CONTENTS

INTRODUCTION

When it comes to working out and gaining muscle, there are a number of moves that can help you increase your muscle mass. While diet is the other part of the equation, you must exercise to ensure you get the results you want.

Ask yourself what you're going after. And, from there, you can create a workout plan that will have you looking chiseled from head to toe! If you're unable to come up with a plan of your own, consider this particular style of workouts that I have developed for myself and other clients, which includes simple workouts for every muscle group in your body with different tips and tricks to maximize your time spent in the gym. For more tips, tricks, vids and live monthly Q & A's, join my Facebook group community at https://www.facebook.com/groups/kratosfpg

But first, let me introduce myself and give you a little about me.

I'm a military veteran who served in the United States Air Force. While serving, I have had the privilege of working around the Commander and Chief of the United States Barack Obama, foreign dignitaries, and other influential people in and around the D.C, Maryland, and Virginia area.

I got into the fitness industry to help people. I know it sounds cliché, but it's the truth! I want to change the fitness industry and make it about people again. What makes me different from everyone else? Passion; My passion for people, my passion for getting people results, and my passion for seeing people evolve into a better, stronger, more confident version of themselves by arming them with tips and tricks I've gained through the years. I've always believed that my job as a trainer isn't just to train people but to motivate and inspire people to move past their perceived limitations.

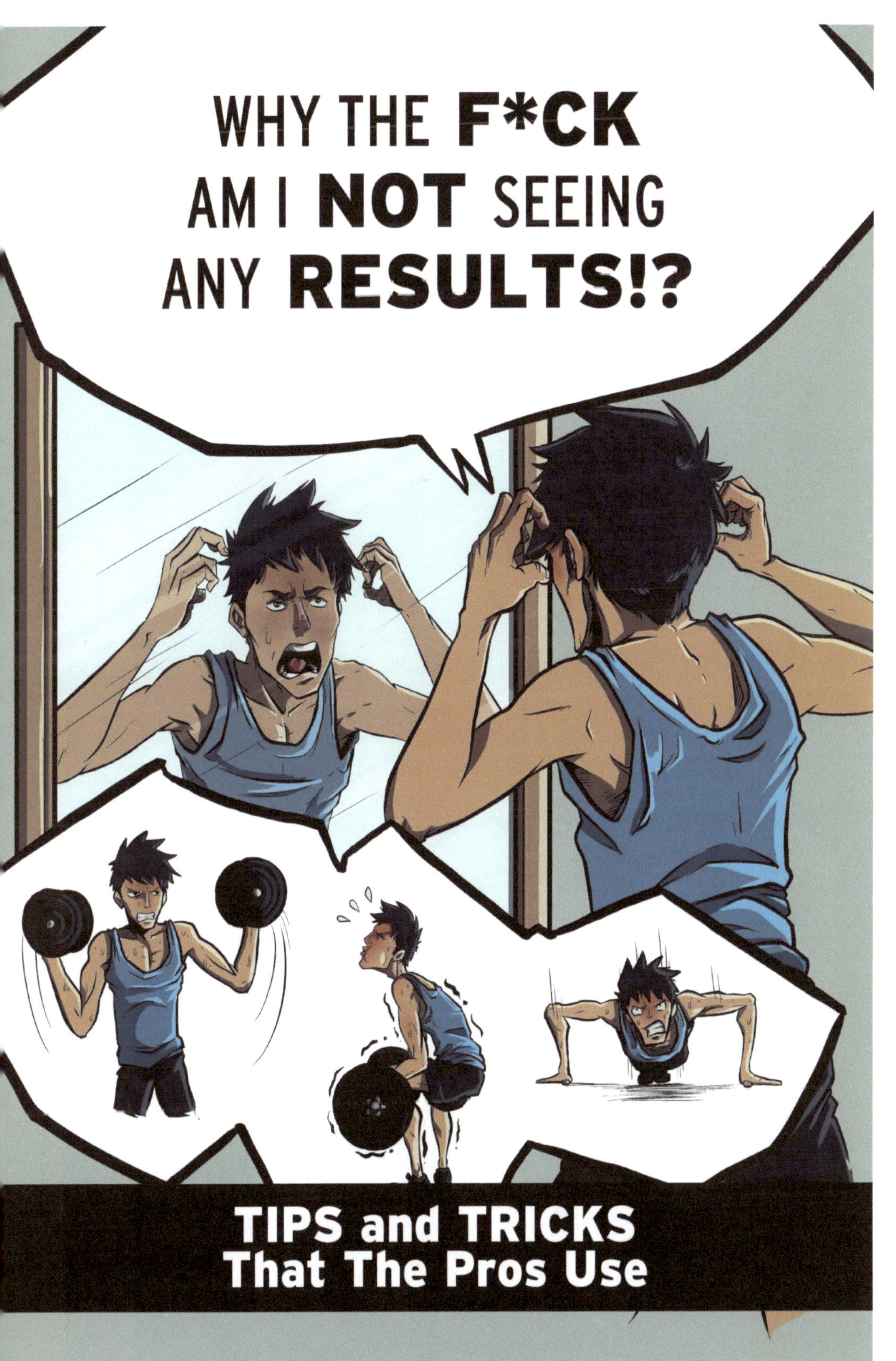

WHY THE F*CK AM I NOT SEEING ANY RESULTS!?
TIPS and TRICKS That The Pros Use

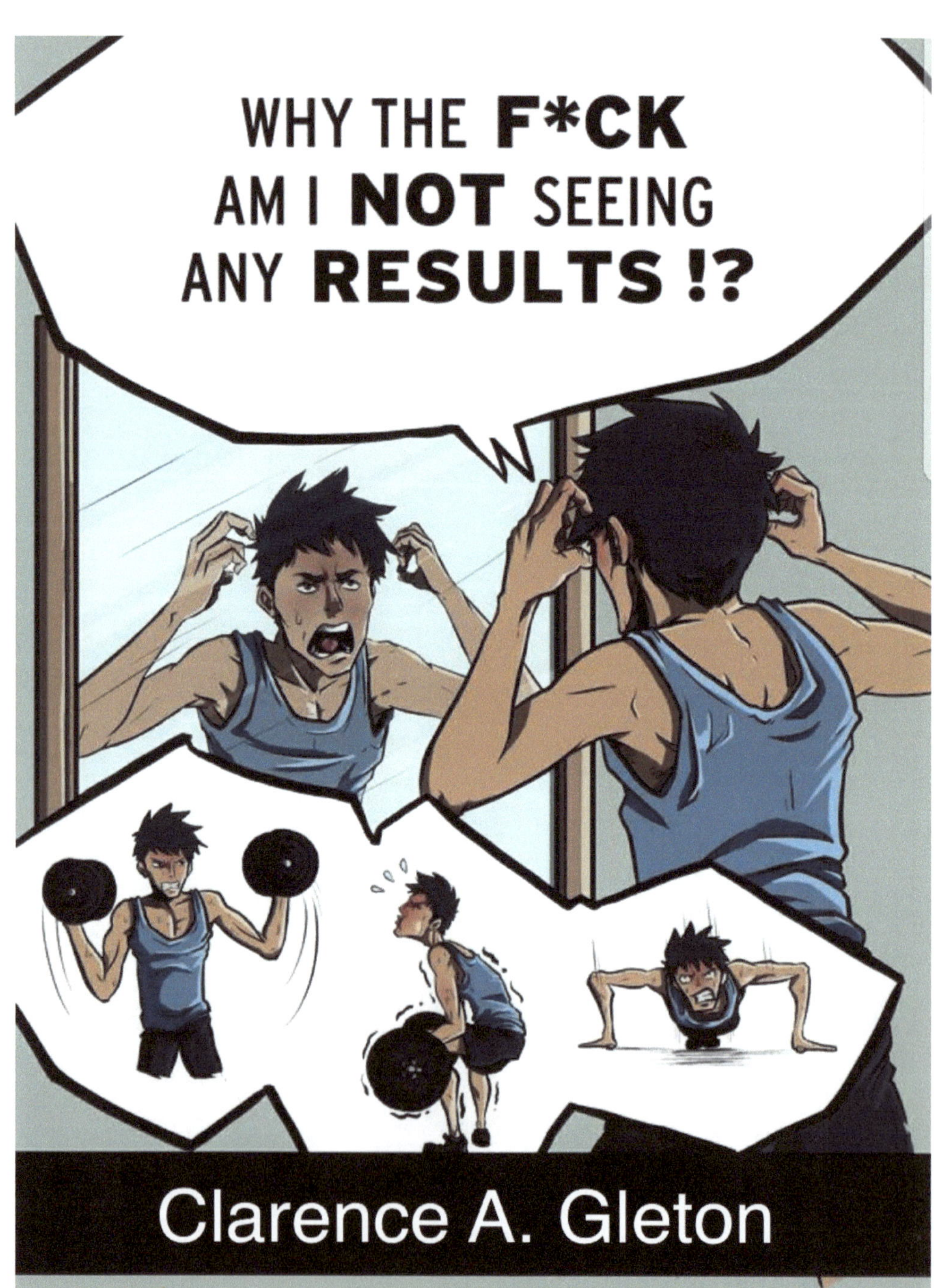

WHY THE F*CK AM I NOT SEEING ANY RESULTS !?
Clarence A. Gleton

Limitations placed upon them by family members, friends, and most importantly, the limitations they placed upon themselves. My background of being an athlete and a military veteran has shown me ways to push myself mentally. Believe it or not, fitness is way more mental than it is physical. If you want change in your life, you have to change the way you think.

At the end of this book will be a sample of a particular high paced training program that combines a number of lifting principles to not only cause you to lose weight by raising your heart rate but also incorporates strength training, endurance training, and hypotrophy. But first, I need to arm you with the tips and tricks to make your workout more effective and efficient.

MOVEMENTS FOR ABS

If you want to focus your workout on your abs, there are three worthwhile exercises that you can do:

- Hanging Leg Raise (front)

- Hanging Leg Raise (side)

- Side Bends (need a dumbbell)

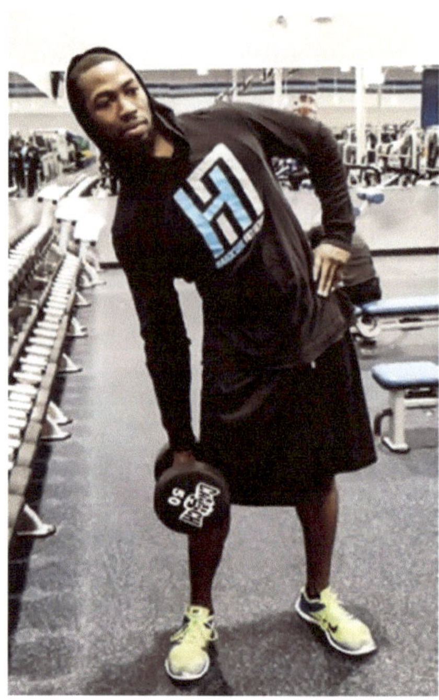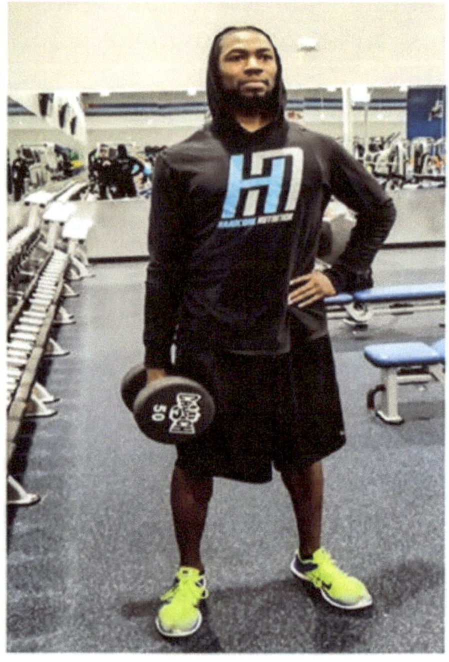

The side bends is a great way to bring your oblique's to the forefront of your core. To the secret to really doing this move to efficiently is to maintain tightness in your core. To engage your core, you want to take a deep breath in and embrace like you're about to get punched in the gut. Often on the top portion of the movement, people tend to over extend to the opposite side which is not called for. Not really needed if you're keeping your core tight throughout the whole movement. High reps is best suited for this great move to really benefit from it.

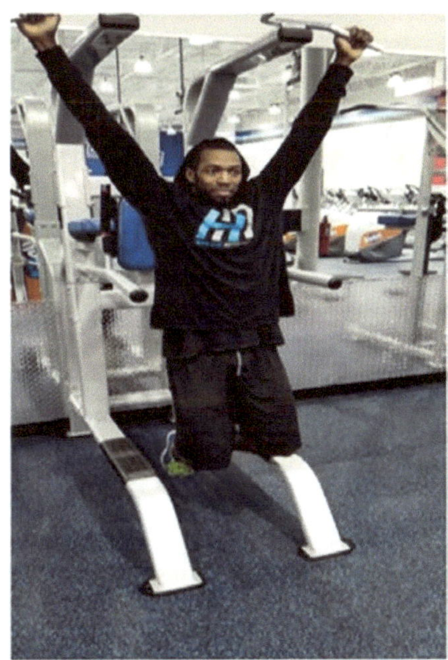
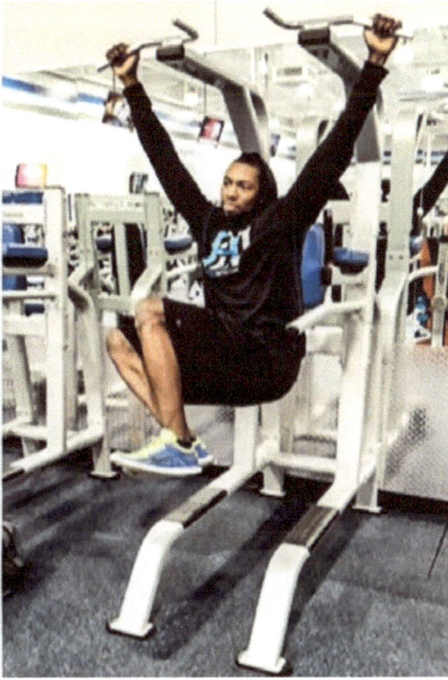

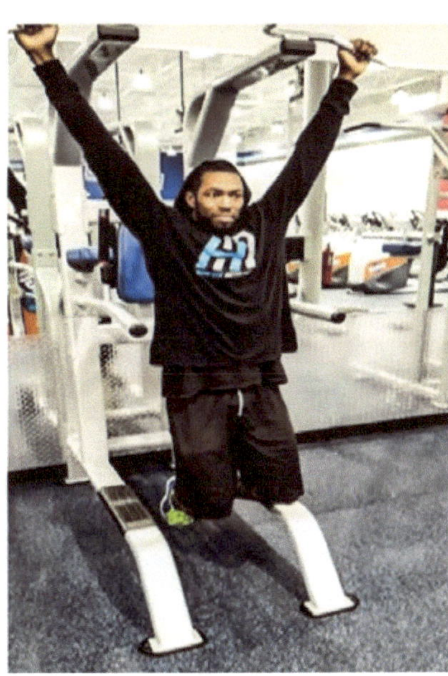
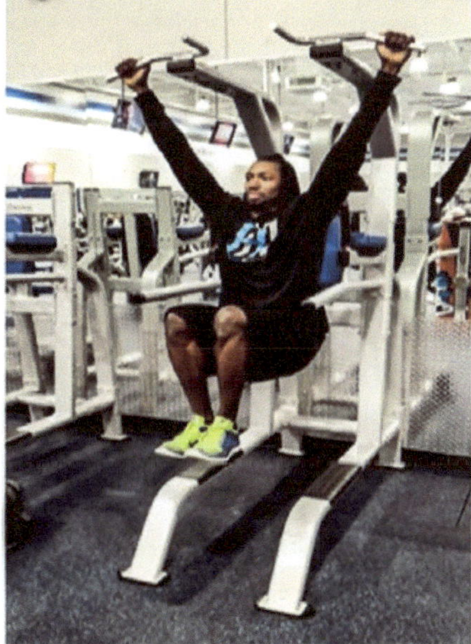

One of my absolute favorites when it comes to core strengthening programming is the hanging leg raise because even while you're hanging there, you are still engaging your core. This being a real simple movement, you start at the bottom of the movement (pictured on the left) and raise your legs (straight or bent as shown in the picture on the right) to the middle and both sides. I typically like high reps with this move (15-20 per side), but if you wanted to turn up the heat by adding a dumbbell (not pictured), then I would suggest 8-12 reps per side.

When it comes to the front hanging leg raise, you have an array of variations to the move. For example, keep the leg straight and bend at your knees. While doing each movement, be sure to keep the core as tightly as you can. You want to ensure there is some tension.

With the side bends, you will need to hold a dumbbell in one hand. Lean to the side – going as far as you can before you start to bend your knee. Slowly come back to the upright position.

MOVEMENTS FOR ARMS

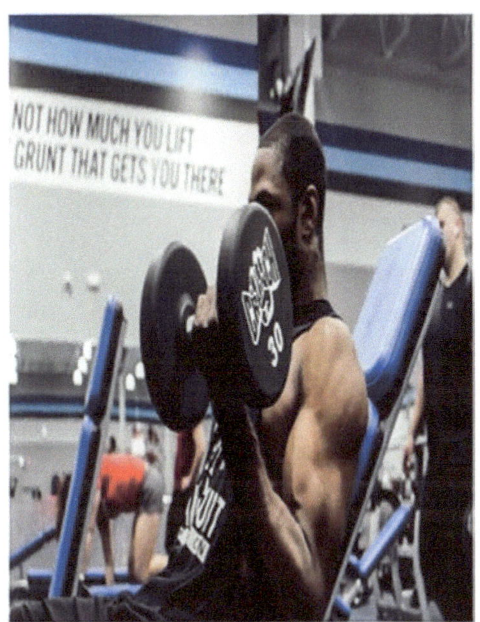

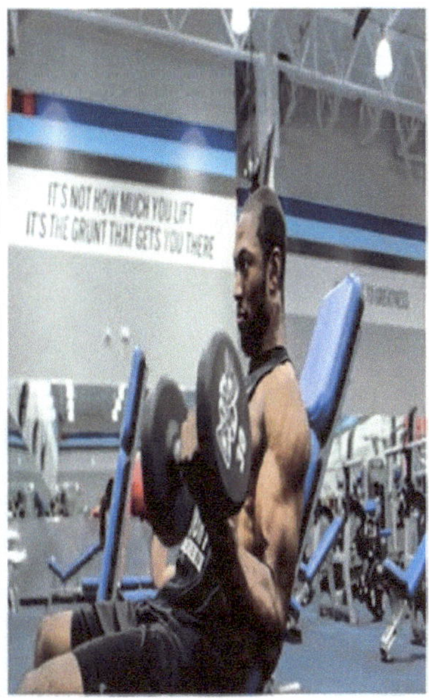

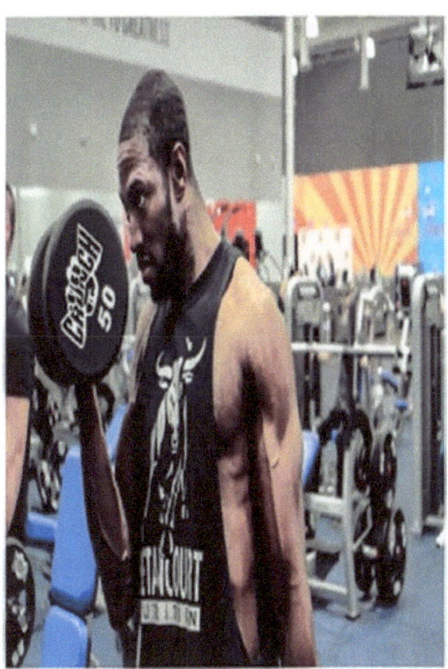

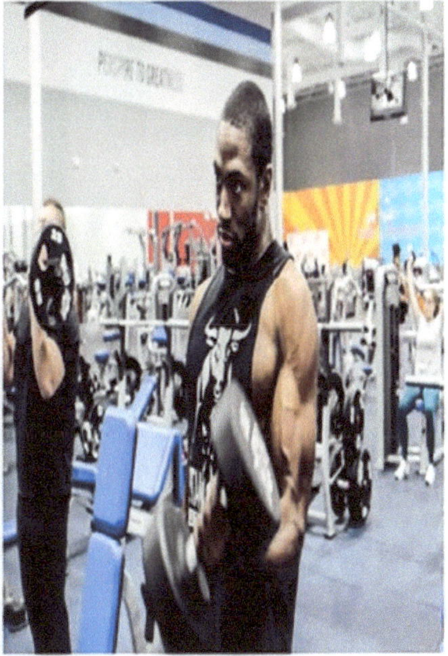

There's no need in reinventing the wheel when the wheel isn't broken. I personally never saw the reasoning or the benefits of what I like to call "Gorilla Curls." You know what these are, you probably saw this in the gym or do it yourself. It looks like someone is beating on their chest with the dumbbells instead of doing a regular curl. With the secrets, I'm about to give you for curls; you will be head above shoulders of everyone else looking to add inches to their mountain tops, otherwise known as biceps.

<u>BICEP SECRET #1:</u> As you are performing the bicep curl (standing or sitting), focus on keeping your elbows as tight to your body as possible. By doing this, you are keeping the tension on the bicep which promotes the tearing of the muscle.

<u>BICEP SECRET #2:</u> Do seated incline curls instead of standing curls. You will sacrifice weight for strength, but the overall payoff is greater. The other thing I love about seated incline curls is that you take your body out of the equation and put all of the focus (where it should be) on the bicep, which will humble you if you're moving a lot of weight standing up.

<u>BICEP SECRET #3:</u> With much lighter weight at the end of your set, squeeze as hard as you can for a count of 3. The reasoning behind this is to force the blood through your veins and expand your bicep muscles for an even bigger pump.

Bicep Exercises

With the standing alternating dumbbells curls, you'll do them in pyramid style training. You'll run the stack or go up the hill or go down the hill. Choose five different sized weights – in increments of five pounds (10lb, 15lb, 20lb, 25lb, etc.) Complete five reps each ending at the heaviest weight for three to four sets with no rest until you've gotten through the last rep on your heaviest weight.

If you want to boost the exercise's intensity, upon reaching the last rep of the heaviest weight, go back down the hill to the lightest weight with no less than three reps each time down the hill. While you do this move, make sure your core is engaged. And, make sure your elbows are near your side.

At the start of the set or near the end, if you decide to go down the hill while you lift the lighter weights, be sure to squeeze your arms at the bottom of the moment. At the top, hold the pose for three seconds.

When it comes to incline dumbbells curls, you'll be using drop sets in all sets. You'll need three sets of dumbbells – light to medium weight. Like above, you want the first part of the reps to squeeze at the bottom with a three-second holding count at the top squeeze movement. The heaviest of the dumbbell should be first, being completed at eight reps. In the second dumbbell set, no more than 10 to 12 reps. In the final dumbbell set (the lighter of the three), you want to do between 12 and 15 reps. Be sure your elbows are kept to your sides during the entire movement.

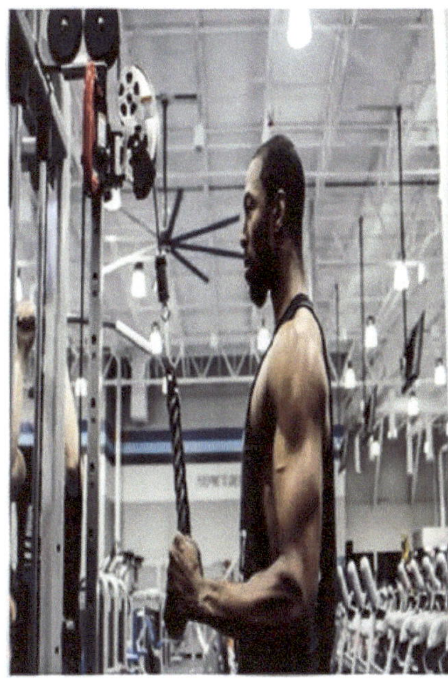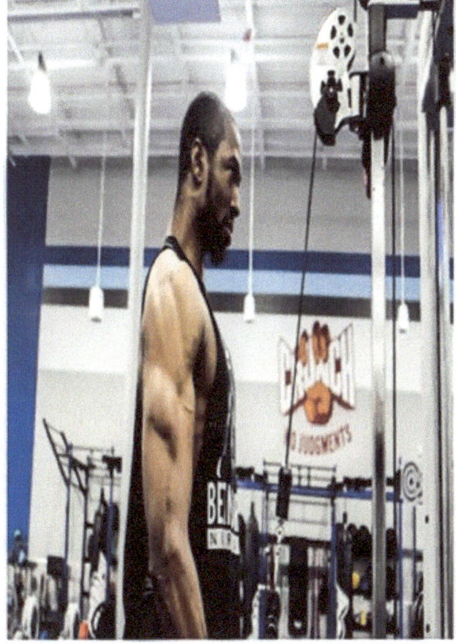

Tricep pulldown's is one that I feel is often incorrectly. Most people go as heavy as they can and use their body weight to help move the weight instead of actually letting their triceps do the work. Imagine you get into a fist fight with a guy and all of a sudden, 3 of his friends jump in the fight to help him out. Unfair advantage, right? That's exactly how it is when people use their body to move the weight instead of the actual muscles that they are supposedly focusing on. Which lead us into one of the main secrets for triceps.

TRICEPS SECRET #1: Don't lean into the weight to move it! Use the muscles you're focusing on! Instead of leaning forward over the weight, stand straight up, shoulders back, chest out as shown in the picture above. The added benefit is that while doing it in this manor, you are also targeting your core by stabilizing you as you move the weight.

TRICEP SECRET #2: Keep your elbows pinned to your side. Think of you elbows as a door hinge. When your elbows are flared out than your door is off the hinges.

TRICEP SECRET #3: Stop parallel to the floor. As shown in the picture on the left, you can see that the forearms are parallel to the floor, not allowing the weight to go all the way back up. When you stop parallel to the floor, you are keeping the tension on the intended muscle, not allowing it to rest or catch its breath before the next full rep.

TRICEP SECRET #4: A little-known secret is to twist your wrists out to recruit more of the triceps into action

Triceps Exercise

The straight bar pulls down and triceps pull down is nearly the same. The only difference is that the straight bar and hand placement needs to be at the end of the bar. While doing this move, be sure you don't go above parallel at the top. While on the bottom, turn your wrists slightly, putting more of the tension on the triceps. Squeeze the muscle while in the movement and hold it for a three-second count.

Special Note: There's no particular rep count here. Just stay above five reps until the lightest weight has been attained.

Cable kickbacks are carried out similarly to the dumbbell kickbacks. This move ensures attention on the triceps. When doing this movement, be sure you note where your elbow is at. You want them parallel to the ground like the triceps. Make sure your forearm is extended, and you twist your wrist to place tension on the triceps.

Other Movement You Can Do:

- Close grip incline bench press

- Skull crushers

- Triceps pull down with rope

- E-Z bar curls or straight bar

MOVEMENTS FOR BACK

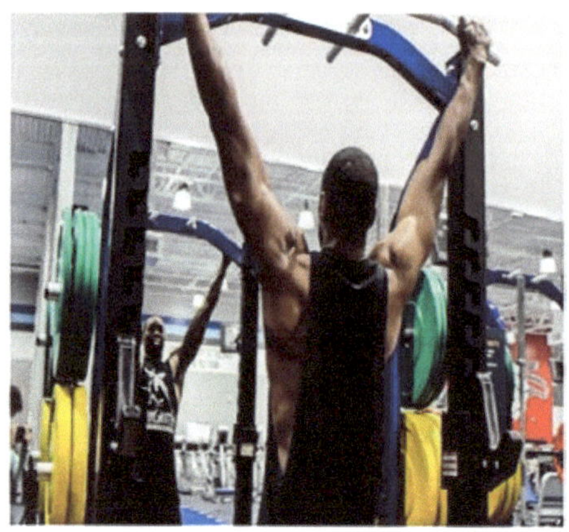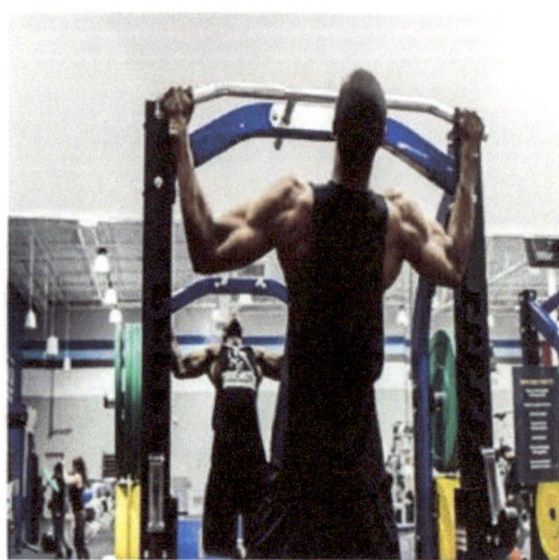

The Pull Up is One of the Kings of back movements. But normally people just pull themselves up (if they can even do one) and go return to the starting position without giving much thought to if they are doing it right. The goal feels the movement in your back, more so in your lats. To make that happen, you have to have a slight lean backwards to engage the lats and get it firing. Don't think of it as bringing your chin to the bar, think of it as bringing your upper chest to the bar. This is a technique that "The Oak" (Arnold Schwarzenegger) used to help grow his back and bring detail really.

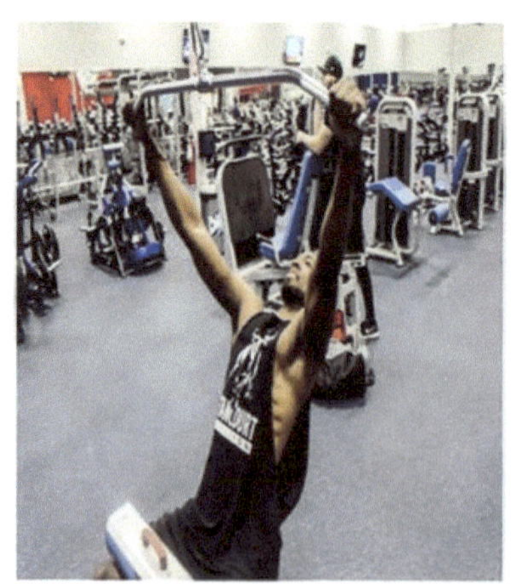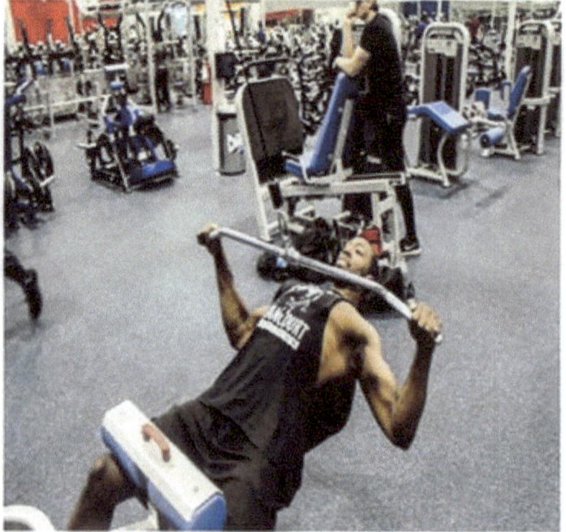

Rather you know it or not ***this isn't the way you should perform the Lat Pulldown***, but its one of those moves that's performed wrong all the time. The Lat Pulldown is similar to a pull-up and should be performed as such. The only difference is that you're sitting down while performing this move. The correct way (shown below) doesn't require you to jerk to perform this move, which I'm sure you have seen on many occasions at the gym. When performed correctly, it's an easy flowing move that really targets your Lats, **IF YOU'RE IN THE PROPER POSITION!**

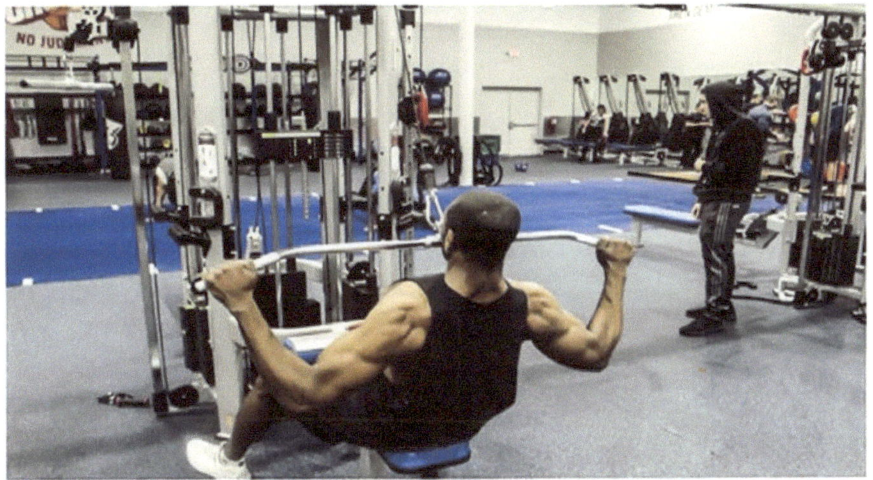

In this picture, you can tell that there isn't much of a lean-to accomplish this move. The goal should be to lean back just enough to engage the focus area which is the Lats.

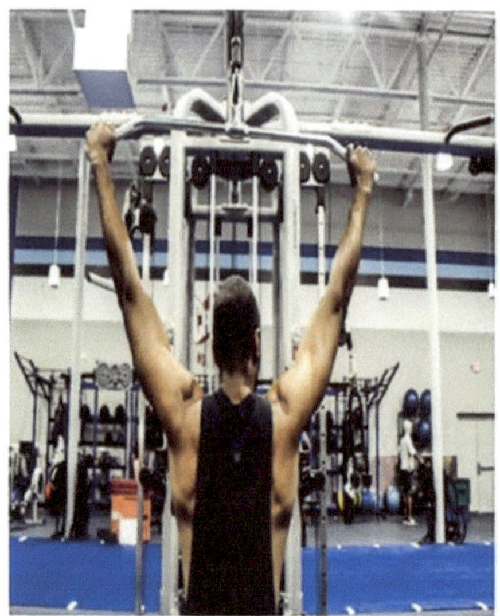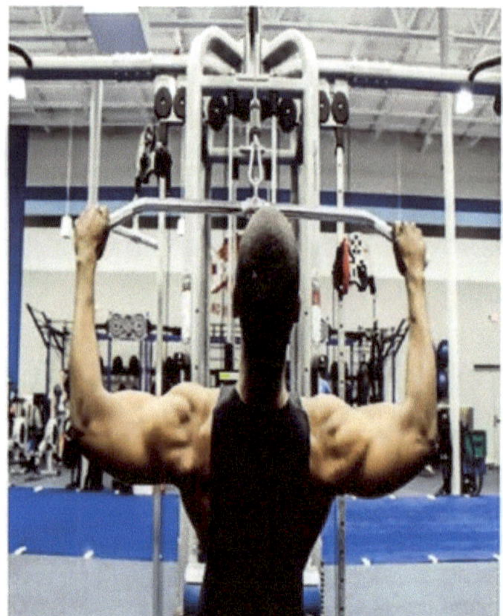

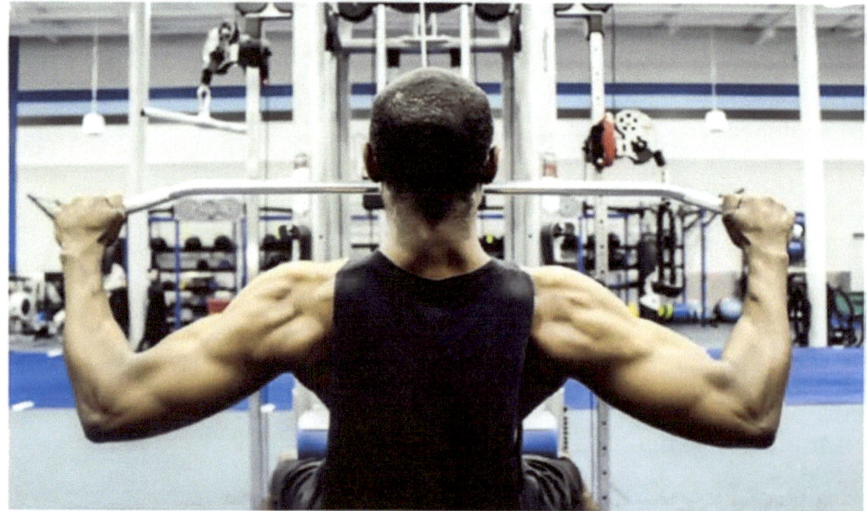

<u>LAT PULLDOWN SECRET #1:</u> Again, this should be a smooth movement from top to bottom, so when you come to the bottom position of this move bring your elbows back. After bringing your elbows back, contract and squeeze your shoulder blades together hard all in one smooth movement. Better yet, try holding it for a count of 3.

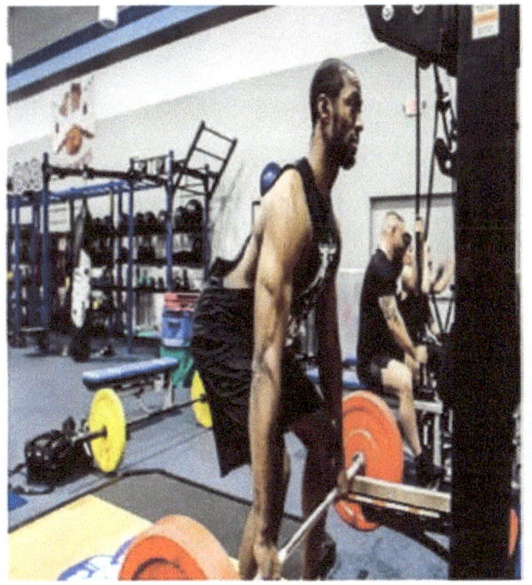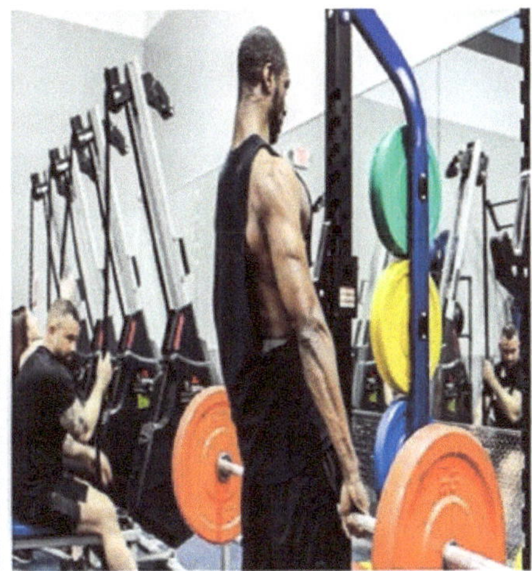

Rack Pulls is a movement that's very seldomly done, which is the reason why I would recommend it for back development. Deadlifts is another great move for back development, but if you have weak points at the top of your deadlift, this is the move that I would recommend. Plus, another great thing about the rack pull is that you keep the tension on your back for the most of the movement. The Rack Pull is similar to the deadlift in all the technique and more; the only difference is that the starting position is raised but right below your knees, recruiting more muscles to complete the movement.

RACK PULL/DEADLIFT SECRET #1: Keep your chest up and back as flat as you can before starting the movement. Retract the shoulders and start to pull like your life depends on it!

RACK PULL/DEADLIFT SECRET #2: Change the way you look at this movement. Instead of pulling the weight, see yourself pushing the ground away.

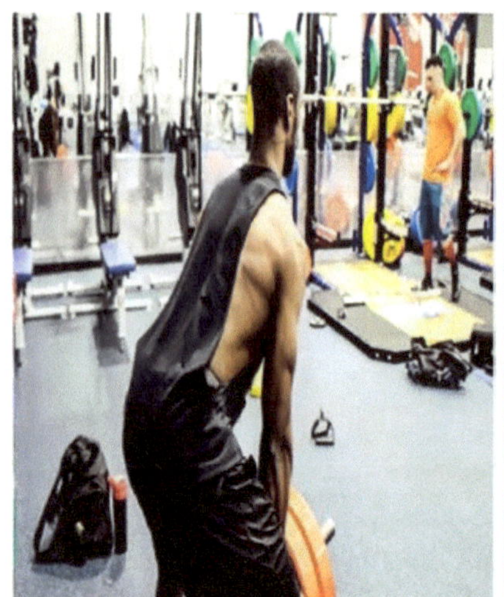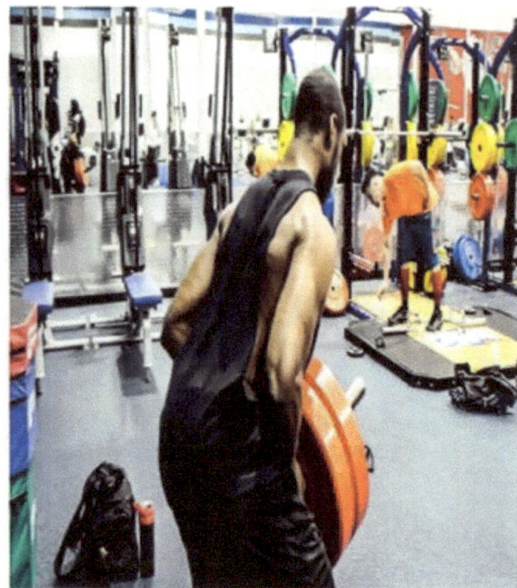

This is another movement that I see a lot of people jurking to move a lot of weight to show how strong they are. If you feel the need to jerk, then it's time for you to A.) Rest or B.) drop the weight.

<u>BACK SECRETS #1:</u> From the bottom position, feel the stretch at the as you let the weight freely hang. When you bring the weight back to the top, keep the elbows tight to the body. By doing this you engage the Lats (which is the muscle that we are targeting anyway).

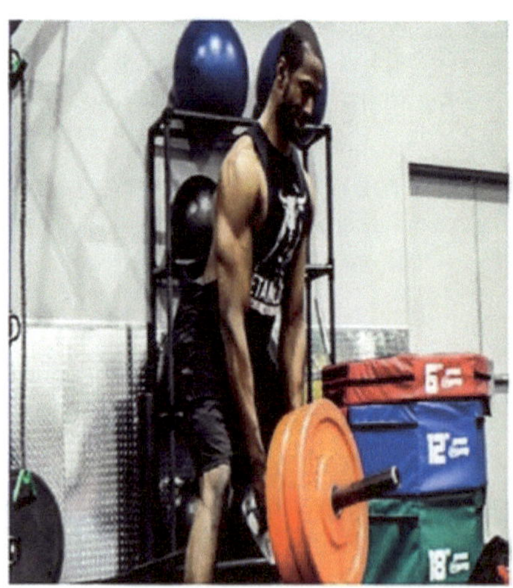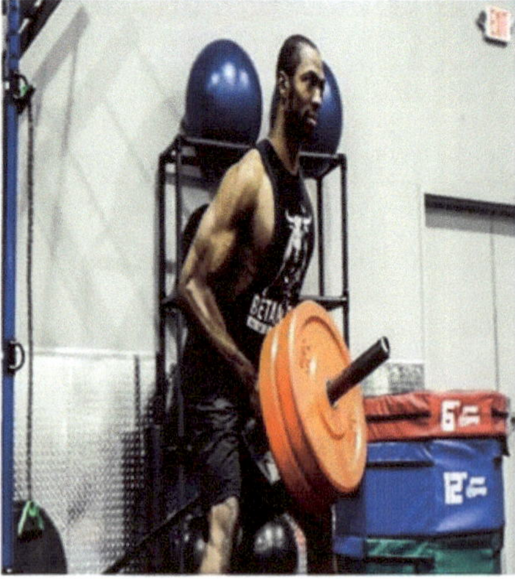

<u>BACK SECRETS #2:</u> It's not always necessary to use 45's. To really get the full effect of this movement use 25lb plates or smaller to get the full ROM (Range of motion). This way you have a more controlled smooth motion throughout the movement.

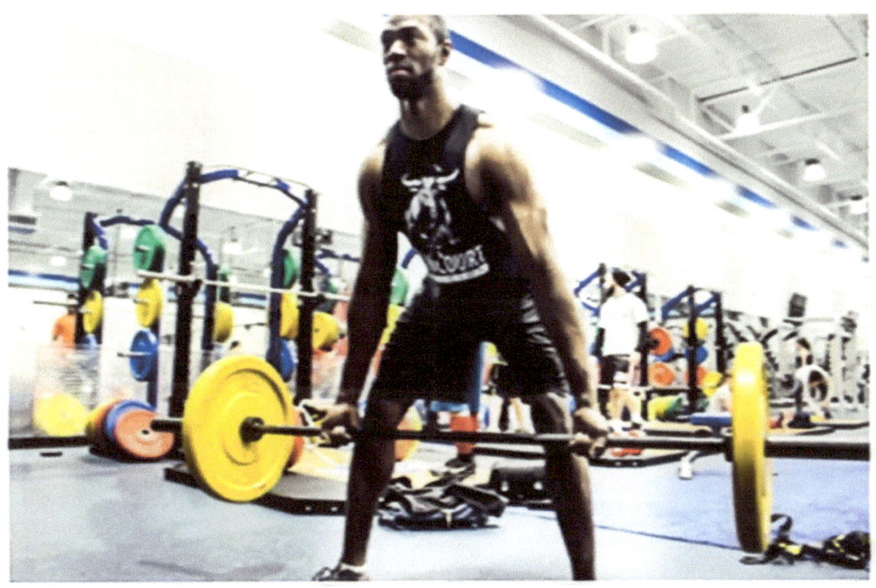

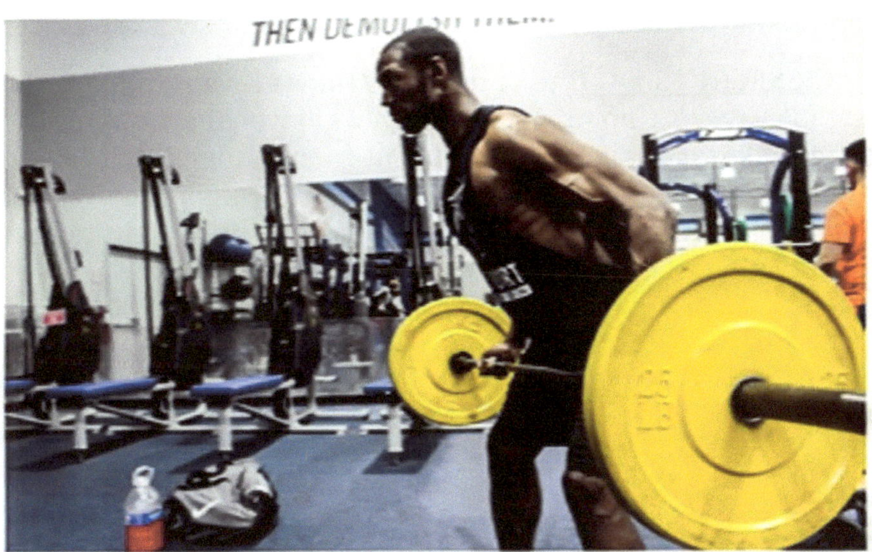

<u>BACK SECRETS #3:</u> To hit the higher and the lower parts of your Lats, you can change the angle of attack by simply bringing the bar or cable above your belly button or below your belly button.

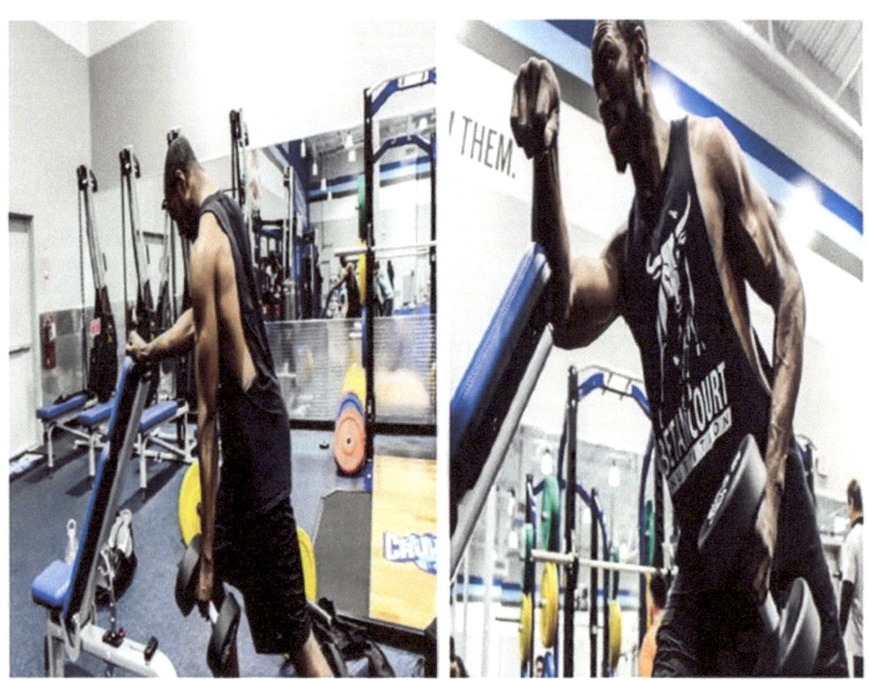

<u>BACK SECRETS #4:</u> One of the main things I want to point out is the way he's holding the weight. I have him holding the weight like this to help prevent him from doing what I like to call "The Lawnmower." It also helps with bringing the weight back more in a semi arc vs. bringing the weight straight up like he's starting a Lawnmower.

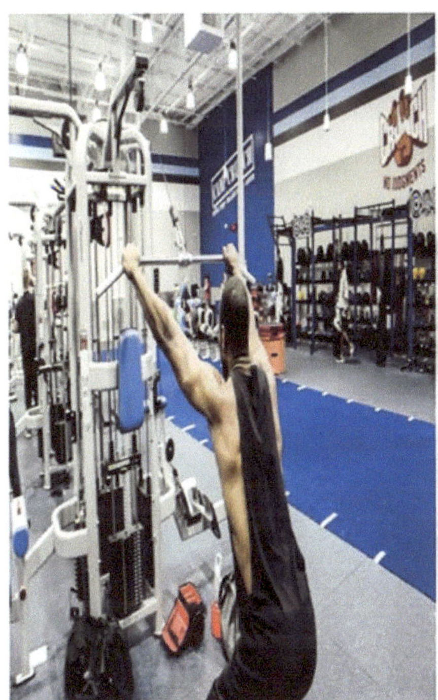 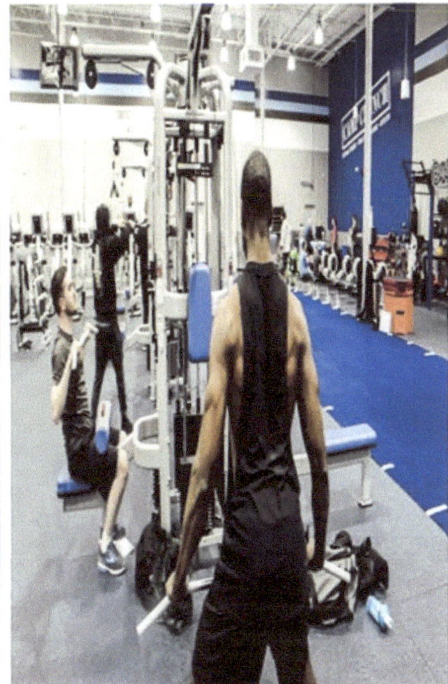

<u>BACK SECRETS #5:</u> One of my favorite moves to tie in the back, best way to do it is to keep your arms semi-locked and pull through contracting the shoulder blades.

Final Thoughts

Back is such a huge muscle which makes it hard to get that mind-body connection, on top of not really being able to feel it. So how do we address this issue? By taking these combined movements slow and squeezing at the top. You have to put your ego to the side and focus on quality reps instead of trying to be like everyone else and move endless amounts of weight with no results. After you learn how the muscle feels when it's doing work, then it's time to start upping the weight slowly.

Make sure you properly warm up your back by doing pull-ups. The problem with this exercise is that the majority of folks fail to do them correctly. Keep in mind that the pull-ups exercise is used through the whole workout, either to pre-exhaust your back or used as a superset in-between the workout's other movement.

How do you do a proper pull-up? Make sure your chest is brought to the bar, slightly arcing your back. When you bring your chest to the bar, you want the elbows to be at the hips. When you do this, the tension is placed on the Lats.

With deadlifts, you never want to go heavy. Instead, use a rather lightweight dumbbell so that you can do eight to 10 reps without much effort. The idea is for you to keep your focus on the technique so that you can use heavier weights later on. Once on the rows, put attention on the shoulder blades, bringing them together and holding it for two seconds.

With the Lat pulldowns, you can do either a wide grip bar or a close grip bar. Or, you can switch up from week to week. This will give your entire back a good workout. You want a drop set for each set by doing heavy weights for eight reps, lowering the weight to complete 10 to 12 reps and finishing the set off with an even lighter weight for 12 to 15 reps.

Special Note: With the weight getting lighter, be sure you squeeze your back for three seconds to ensure the muscles get blood.

Other Movements You Can Do:

- Cable Rows

- Close Group Lat Pulldown

- Smith Machine Rows

- Smith Machine Deadlifts

MOVEMENTS FOR CHEST

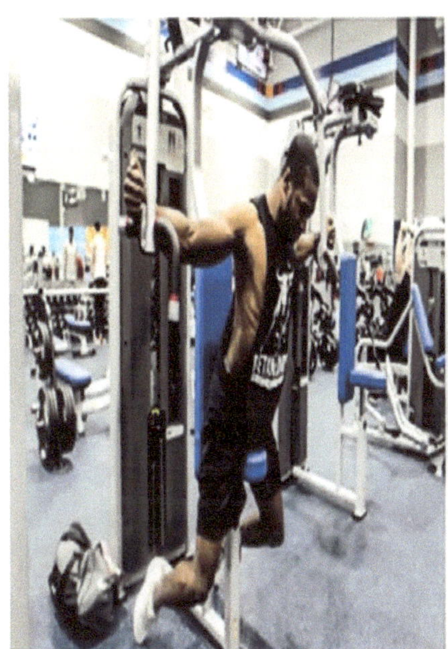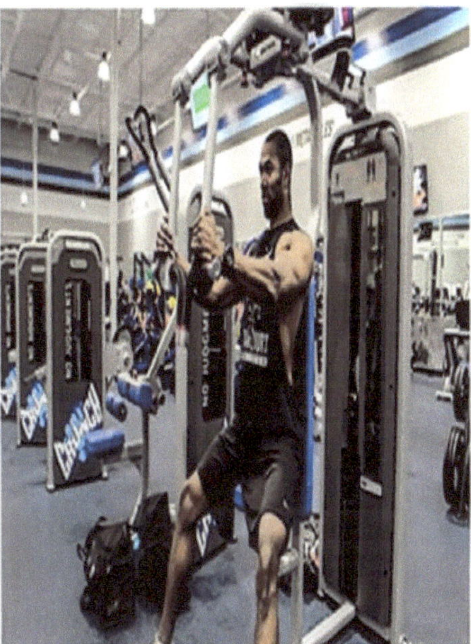

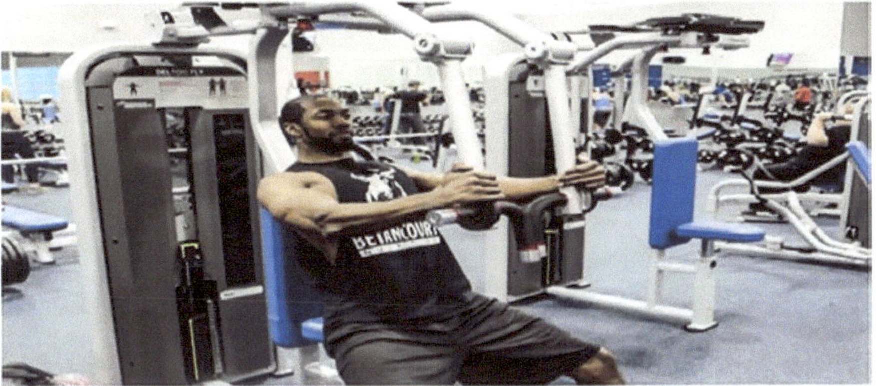

All three of these pictures are of the same movement but executed differently. Top left, the butt is pushed to the back of the seat while leaning forward targeting the upper pecs. The top right, the move is completed the regular way targeting the middle pecs, and the bottom picture the butt is pushed up to the edge of the seat with the upper back pressed against the backboard targeting the lower pecs. This is an excellent move to not only warm up your pecs, but also to pre-exhaust the pecs. Have you ever wondered why your chest isn't sore after completing a grueling chest day? You've failed to pre-exhaust your chest. Add this to the beginning of your chest day completing 10 reps per position without rest focusing on holding and squeezing at the top of the movement in a slowly controlled manor.

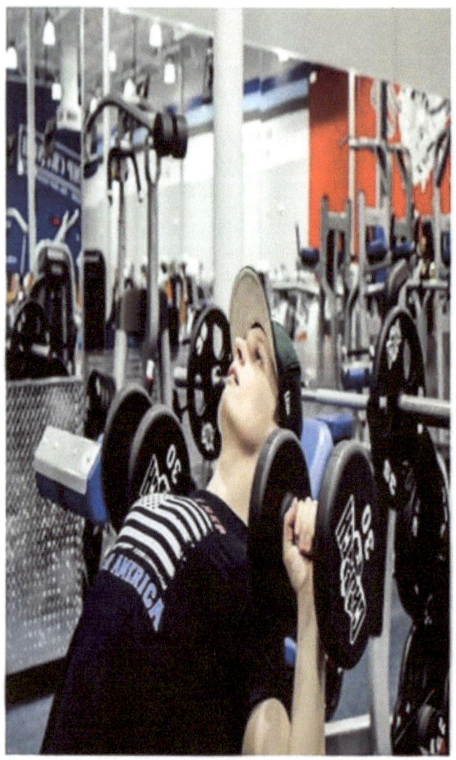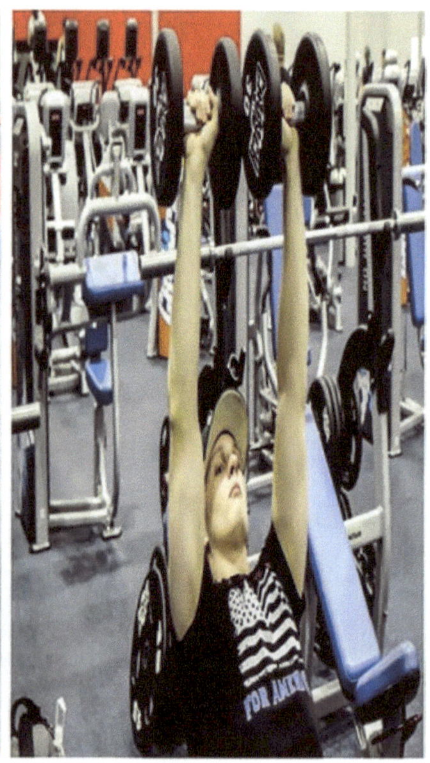

<u>CHEST SECRETS #1</u>: One of the biggest reasons why people are not sore after a grueling chest workout is because they don't know how to activate their chest. The secret is to contract your shoulder blades together when you are on the bench, flat or incline. When you contract your shoulder blades together, you push your chest up which places it in prime position to be activated throughout the movement.

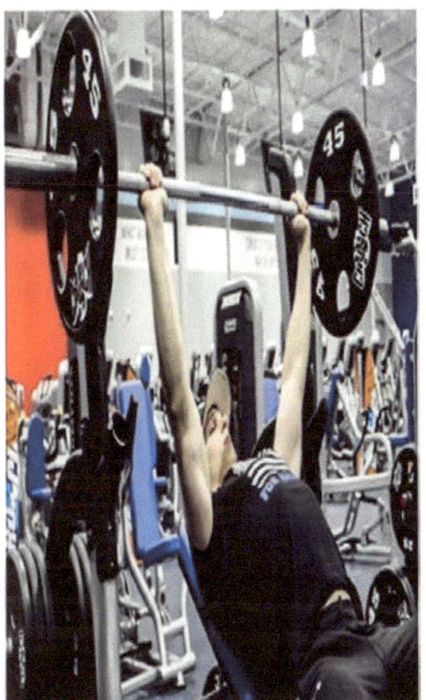 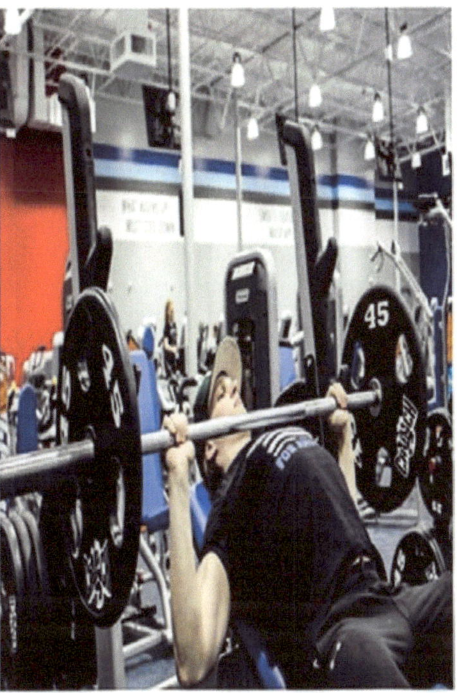

<u>CHEST SECRETS #2:</u> Another main focus when it comes to training chest is form. Don't flare out your elbows as you lower the weight. By doing this, you take the tension off the intended muscle (which is the chest) and place it solely on the shoulder joints. Many people are guilty of this and do it on a regular. Instead, bring your elbows in at a 45degree angle. At A 45degree angle, you are now in a power position to push the weight since this is also a power movement.

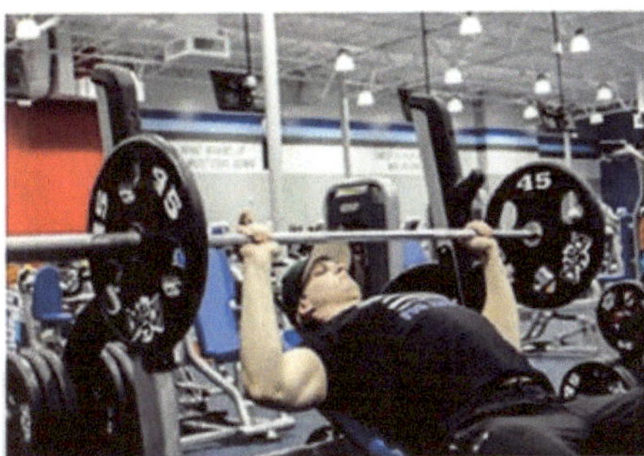 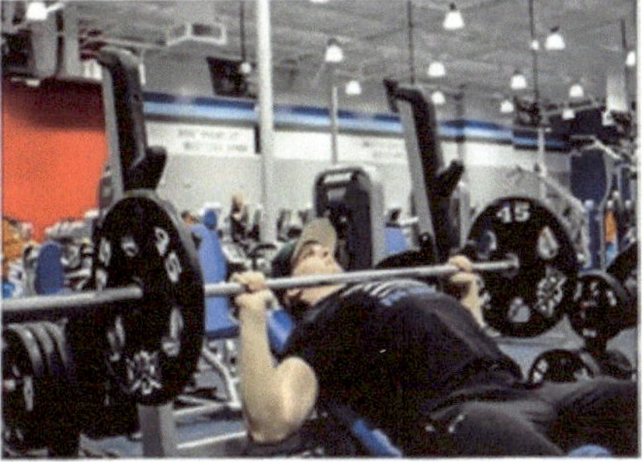

CHEST SECRET #3: Another misconception is how far down you should go on a bench press. Depending on your stature and shoulder health, 90degress should suffice. Per all the textbooks 90 degrees is an optimal to achieve your goal of muscle activation. Now from a more practical standpoint, again depending on shoulder health, going past 90degrees puts your shoulders in a comparable position that can very much cause shoulder issues or damage. If you have good shoulder health with no issues, you should stop right above the chest.

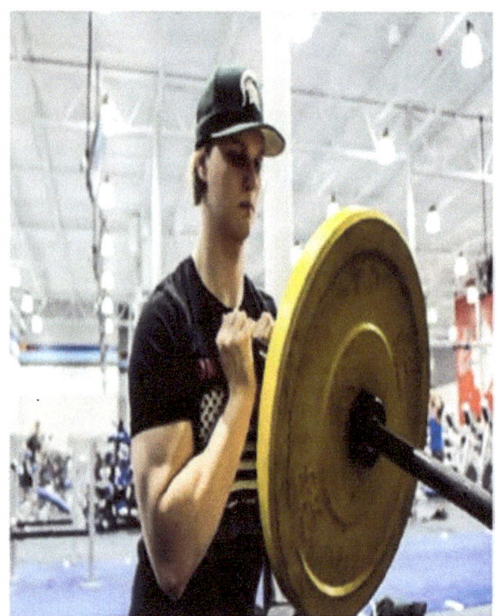
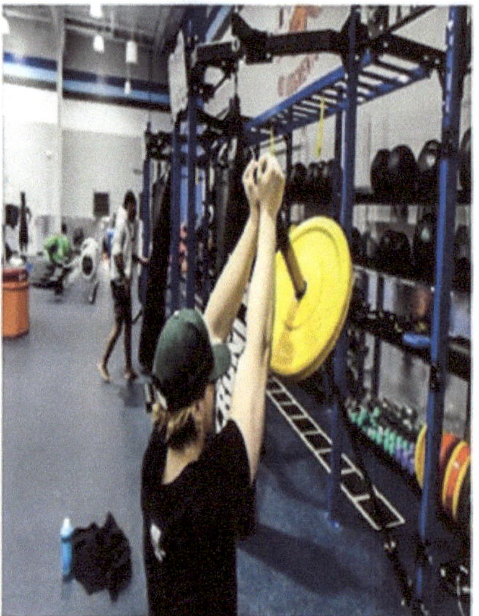

CHEST SECRETS #4: Another major issue I see is lack of upper chest development, mainly because everyone puts so much stock in the flat bench press, which there's nothing wrong with. But if the goal is to achieve the overall astatic look like the great Arnold or "The Myth" Sergio Oliva, then we need to put more focus on the upper chest, which is one of the hardest muscles t bring up. With this move pictured above, focus on keeping your elbows tight and squeezing at the top of the movement. Pick a weight that you can fail at between 8-12 reps.

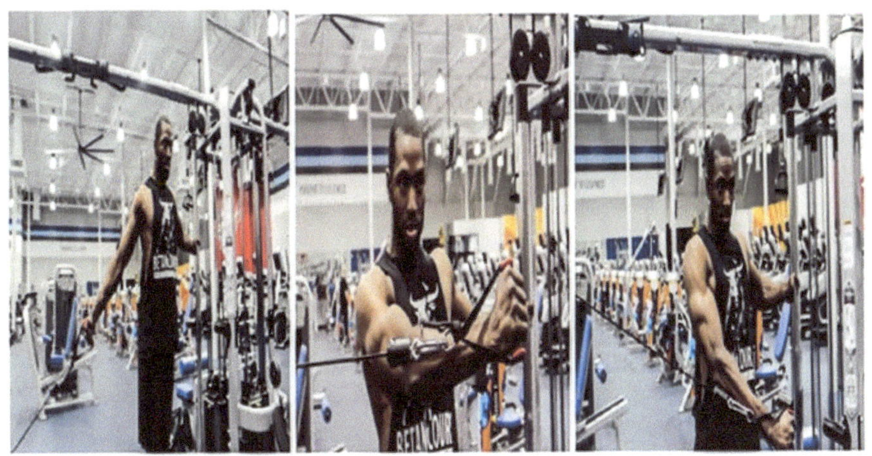

CHEST SECRETS #4: Many people do the cable flies which is an excellent move, but the way they execute it is flawed in my belief. The tendency to load up on weight and position themselves to damn near kiss the floor is unproductive. If done right, by the time you knock out your main movement (The Big Three-Bench, Squat & Deadlift), everything else should be focused on contracting the muscle. Which is why in the three pictures above, the cable fly is done unilaterally or, one side at a time to maximize the contraction (by squeezing the pec), tightening of the core, and focusing on the weak and strong side alike.

CHEST SECRETS #5: By hitting the cables from a high-point (upper pecs), mid-point (middle and outer pec), and low-point (lower pec) without rest is a great cherry on top to end your chest day. By burning out your pecs by doing high reps with the 3count hold and squeeze.

The incline bench press should have a moderate to heavy weight on it for eight to 12 reps. But, the decline machine press should have low weights on them. With the initial five reps, make slow, controlled movements for five seconds at the top of the movement (this means your arms are extended and in a locked position). Be sure you squeeze hard to force the blood to go through your pecs.

Upon finishing the fifth rep, do another 10 reps quickly at a controlled pace for 15 total reps. You also want to do two drop sets in increments of10 pounds until you cannot do anymore. Be sure you alternate each week between incline bench press with moderate light weights for 15 reps and decline press machine for moderate to heavy weights for 15 reps. Alternate with shoulder height crossovers, low cable crossovers, and higher cable crossovers.

Other Movements You Can Do:

- Decline Bench Press

- Decline Dumbbell Press

- Incline Dumbbell Press

- Pec/Dec Machine

MOVEMENTS FOR LEGS

Squats is the **KING OF LEG MOVEMENTS!** The thing that people struggle with most when it comes to squats is that a lot of people have bad form. Which, of course, leads to bad experiences with squats. So, here's the secret to performing near-perfect squats; **CONSTANT STRETCHING!** The more flexible you are, the better you squat. With that said, here are a few things you can do to help open up your hips to increase your flexibility and better your squats.

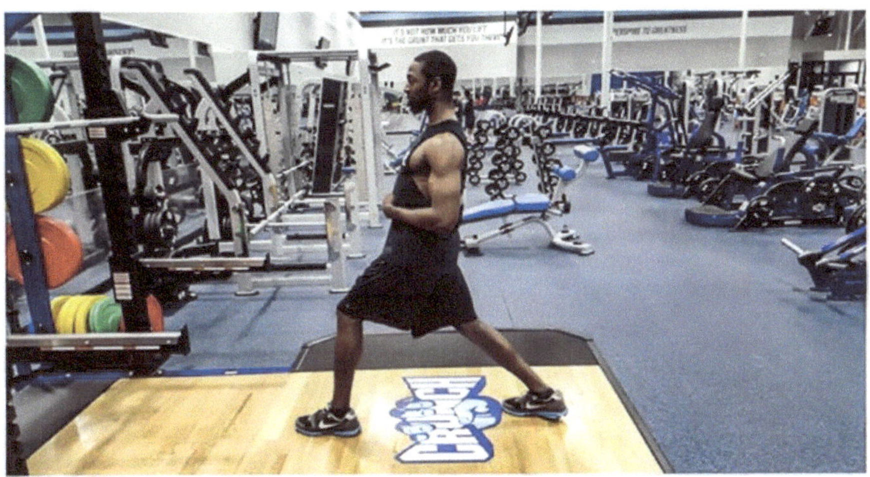

In this position, keep your back heel on the ground and push your hips forward and hold for 15-30 seconds and switch sides. To add more to this stretch, twist to the opposite side of your lead leg with the same hand to help loosen your lower back. Just like in the picture below.

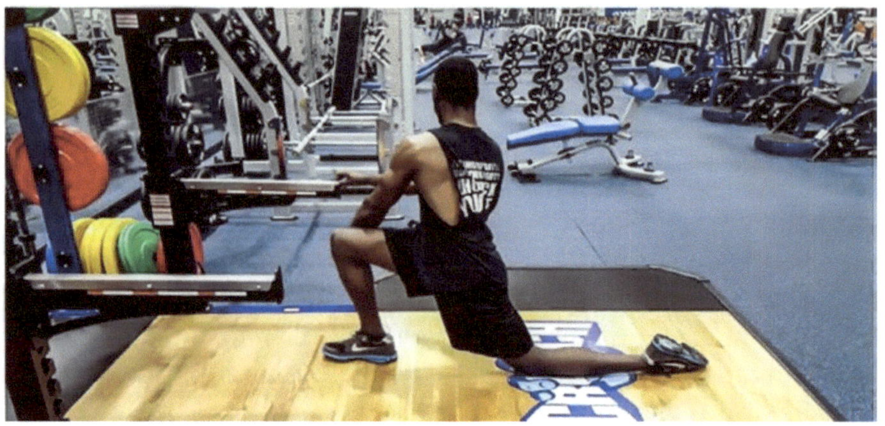

Essentially the same stretch as above but on the ground. In this stretch push your hips forward.

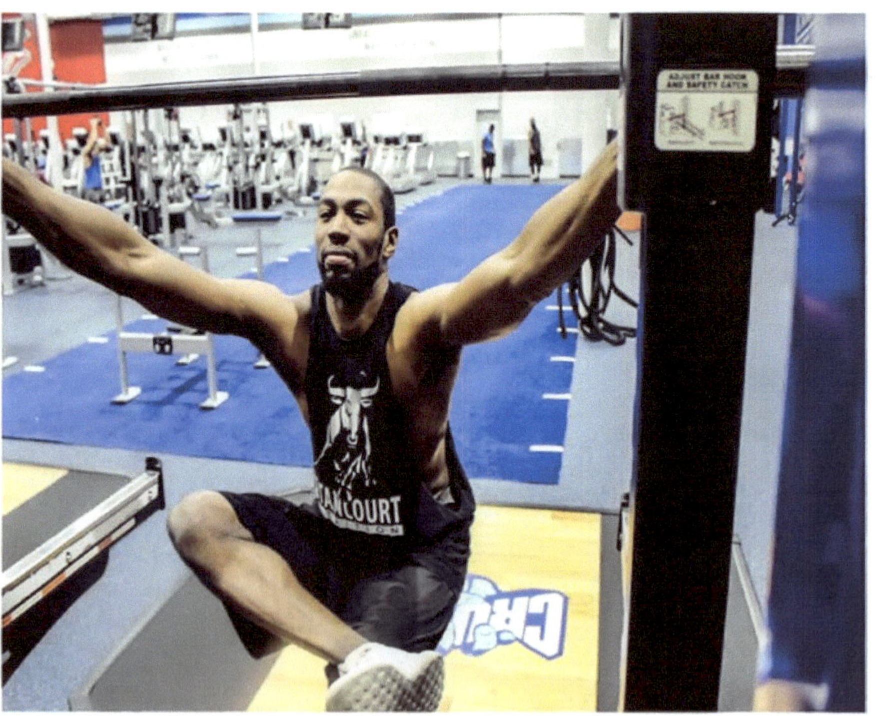

The "Figure Four" stretch is a great stretch to open your hips and to prepare you for the squat. Go as deep as you can to utilize the stretch really.

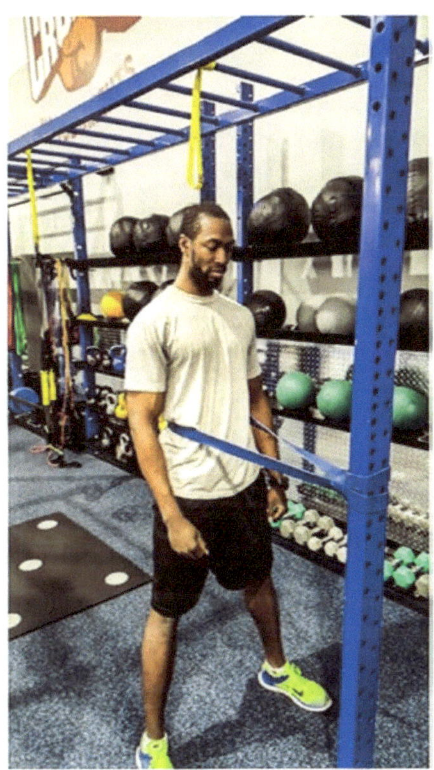 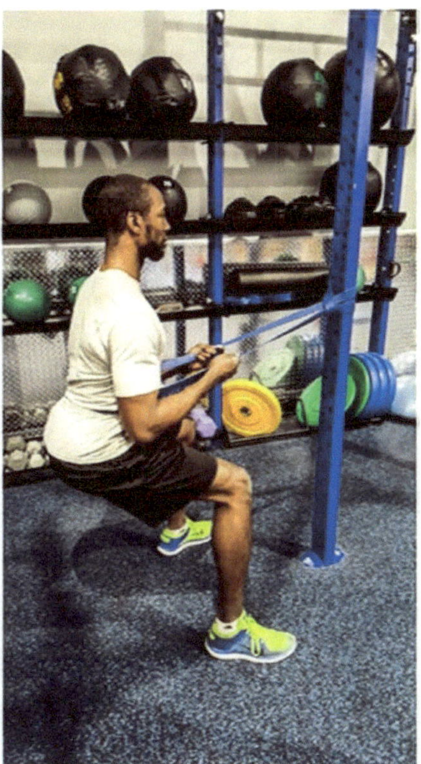

Since I started training, I've noticed how a majority of my clients had a hard time feeling comfortable sitting back on their hips as they squat. Try doing this before squatting for a few months to help you feel comfortable sitting back on your hips.

Now that we got the ways to better your squat let's get into the good stuff.

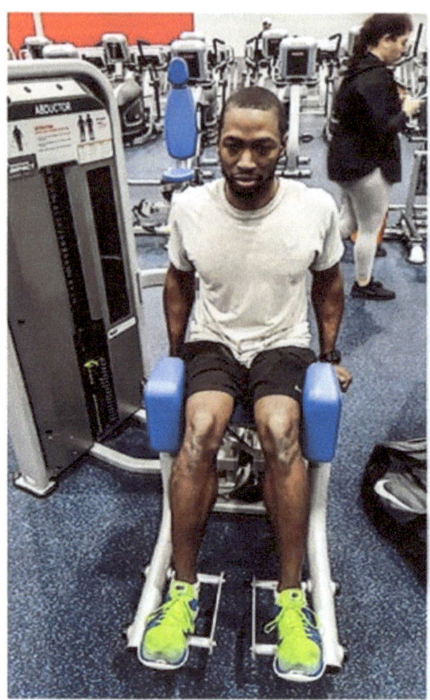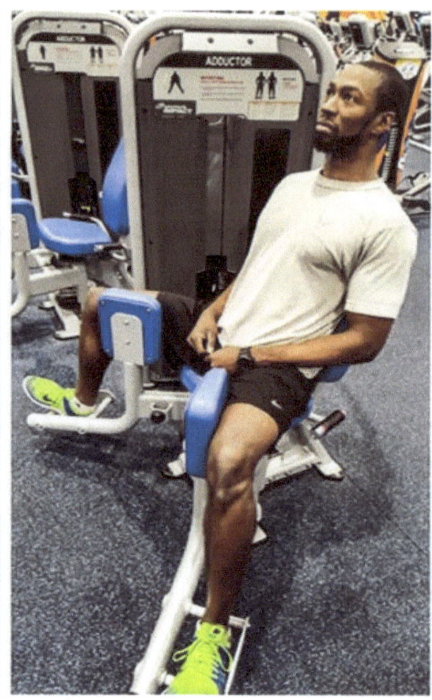

The abductor and adductor machine is a great warm-up for your biggest lift which is the squat. Also, it's a move that a lot of people forget about when it comes to bettering their squat. By using these machines here, it will prevent your knees from clapping or what I like to call the "Bambi" when going down to the bottom and to the top of the squat.

ABDUCTOR AND ADDUCTOR SECRET: I would suggest super setting both movements together doing high reps. But the twist on this movement is holding the first half of your reps for 3 seconds (one one thousand, two one thousand, three one thousand). While holding the first half of your reps (10-12 each machine) focus on squeezing your legs and butt to get the maximum effect of the movement.

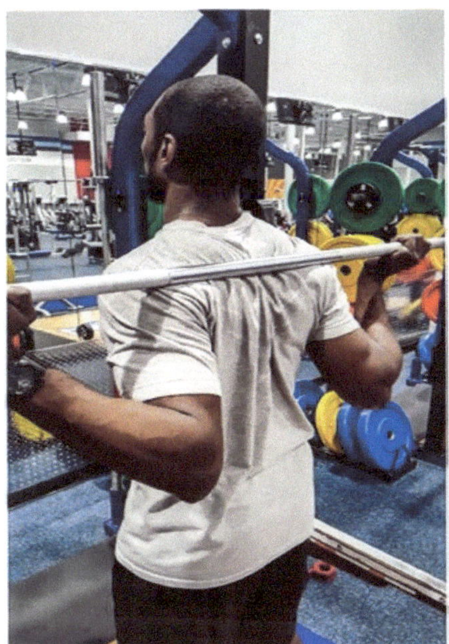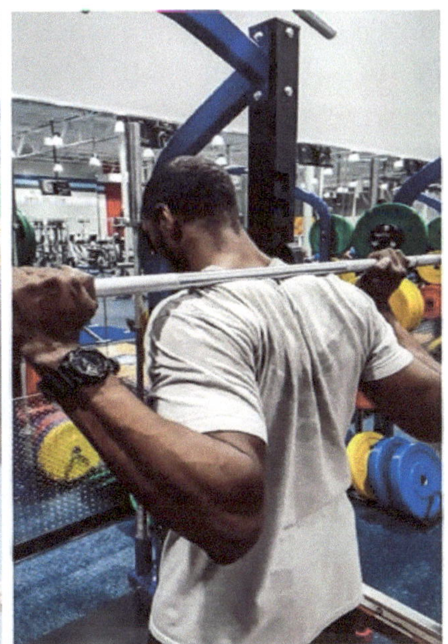

Now that we went through some stretches and proper warm-ups for the squat, the next big thing is figuring out the placement of bar that works best for you. By me being a taller individual, I'm more comfortable with the high bar which is the picture on the right. But I would suggest trying out both the low bar pictured on the left and the high bar to see which one feels more comfortable to you.

SQUAT SECRET #1: While looking at the pictures above, notice how tight my hands are. Bringing in your hands as tight as you can you force your body to stay tight while performing the squat.

SQUAT SECRET #2: While keeping your hands tight you also force your elbows down. This really comes in handy while going to the top position of the squat, giving you more of that push that's needed to finish out the move when you start to hit that wall.

SQUAT SECRET #3: Squeeze your shoulder blades together to help keep your chest up. What tends to happen when people squat is that coming from the bottom position to the top position, the chest drops and the butt starts to rise before the chest. Causing the focus of the movement to shift from the quads and glutes to the lower back instead of keeping the focus on the muscles just mentioned. I don't need to tell you, but another reason people don't like to perform this move is because it causes lower back pain. Know you can understand why and where the pain is coming from. Ideally, you want your body to move as one back to the top of the movement.

Combining these 3 secrets in combination with the stretches and mobility work will do wonders for your squat. The more you squat, the more you will become comfortable and the deeper your squat will be.

Final Thoughts- Before moving on, I would like to dispel some popular "Bro Science" beliefs that deals with squats like "Ass To Grass" or "ATG." Everything has its place, but "ATG" should not always be the goal. Always aim to break 90 degrees. Very rarely do you see anybody squat big weights going "ATG." If you're shorter in stature, it may be more applicable to go "ATG" after mastering 90 degrees than it is for a taller individual (like me) to "ATG." Again, everybody's body is different, but the biggest issue is when people go "ATG," and their knees go way past their toes which shifts the tension and focus more so on the knees which, again, another reason why people don't like performing this movement.

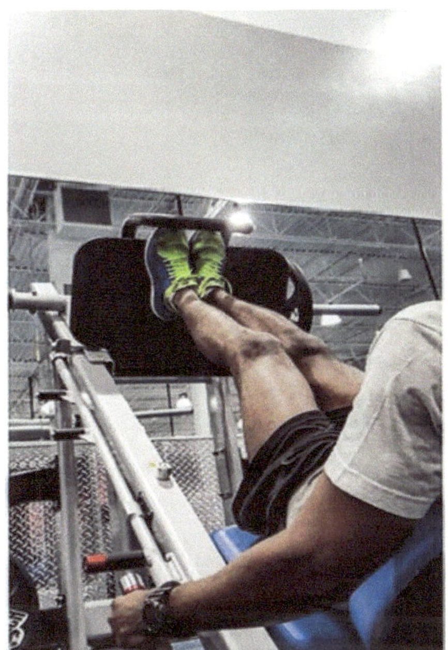 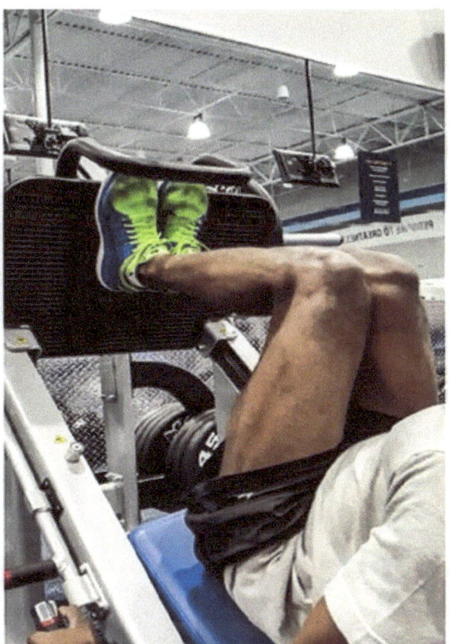

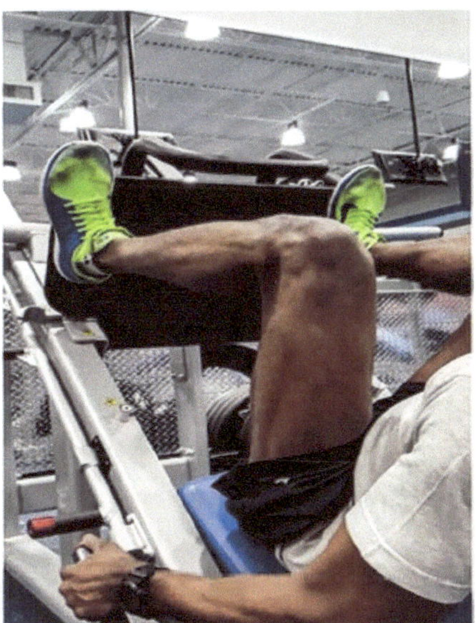 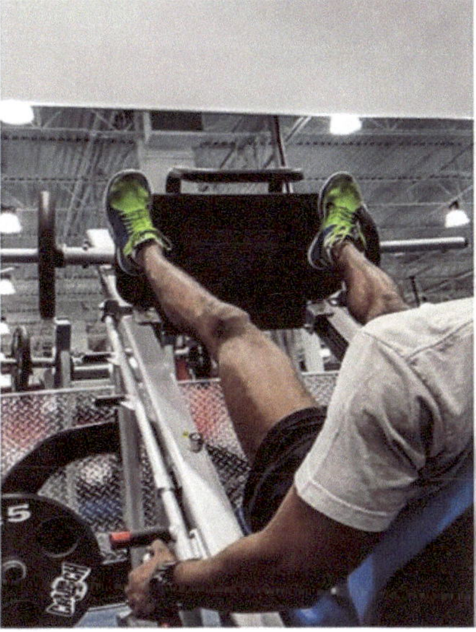

To force my quads to grow, I love super setting this with squats which by the way is already tough enough by itself but well worth its weight in gold. Just a word of caution if you do this super set, don't be in such a rush to go from the squat to the leg press and don't be in a rush to get up afterwards as well. If you're squatting heavy weight after you rack it, make sure you have your barring's before you move on, or you'll be laying on the ground waiting to come to. Even after you complete the leg press afterwards, catch your breath to ensure you won't end up on the ground. Trust me; you'll be glad you did.

LEG PRESS SECRET #1: To focus on the outside of your quads do the leg press with your feet together.

LEG PRESS SECRET #2: While doing leg press with your feet together, focus on not letting your knees move around due to weight

LEG PRESS SECRET #3: KEEP YOUR ASS PLANTED ON THE SEAT! When descending, I've noticed a lot of people going too far which, again, takes the tension off the quads and places it on the lower back causing pain when finished. Go down just before your butt come off the seat to keep the tension where it needs to be, on your quads!

LEG PRESS SECRET #4: Wide leg press focuses on the inner part of your legs to complete the sweeping look everyone wants for their legs. Also for both close and wide stance leg press, I typically like to keep my feet high on the platform, but play around to find the right foot position that works best for you and really targets the quads.

Final Thoughts- Pairing both the squat and leg press, if done properly, will exhaust and fatigue your legs which is the goal. Because we are on our feet all day every day, we must really push our leg training almost to the brink of overtraining for our legs to respond. That is of course, if you're not blessed with great genetics to whereas it doesn't take much for your legs to grow.

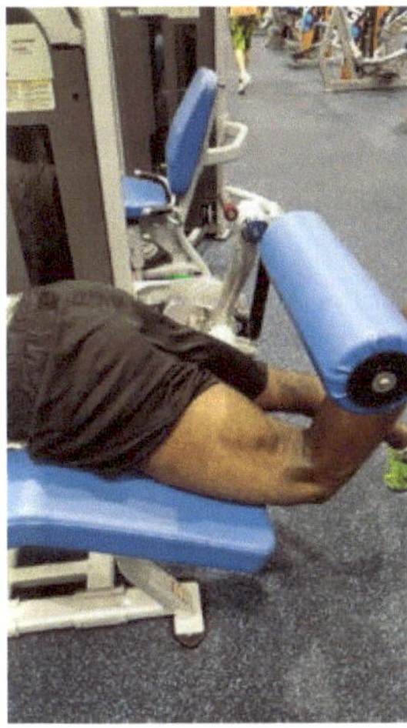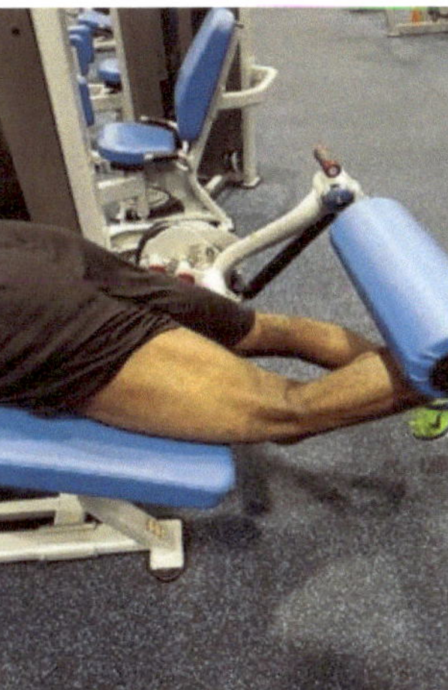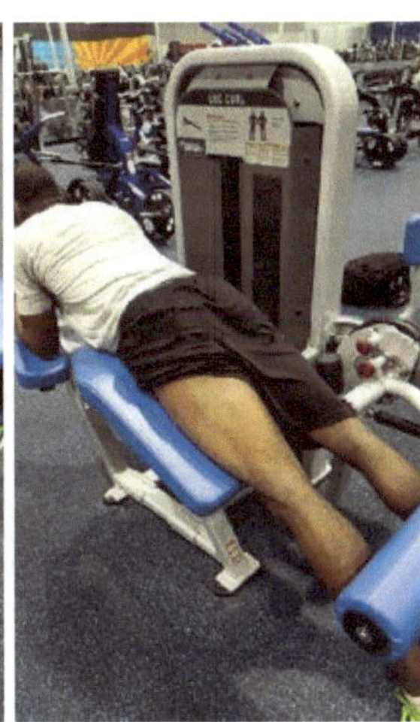

I personally like the lying leg curl as opposed to the sitting leg curls because I can feel it more. Which is more important, the feel of the muscle doing the work.

LEG CURL SECRET: You can't have great legs without great hamstrings! The picture shows three positions of the leg curl for a reason, top, middle and bottom position. The key to great hams is keeping that muscle under constant tension. At the top hold for a 3 count (one one thousand, two one thousand, etc…) hold in the middle for another 3 counts, then finish out the move. While holding for the 3 counts, squeeze hard to force the blood through the veins to expand the muscle. If you're doing 8 reps, hold the first half then rep out the rest to get the full effect.

The key workout for legs is the leg squats, mainly because it incorporates a number of muscles – ankle flexion, knee flexion and hip flexion. The squats are a great movement for the legs. With the 5x5 training principle, your legs become more powerful.

Be sure the leg extensions are done using light to somewhat heavyweight, with five reps held in the up position for three seconds (squeeze the muscle). Finish the remainder of the reps in a precise manner.

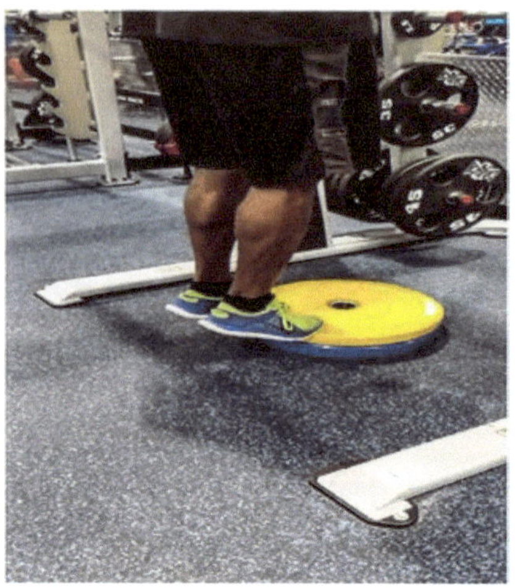 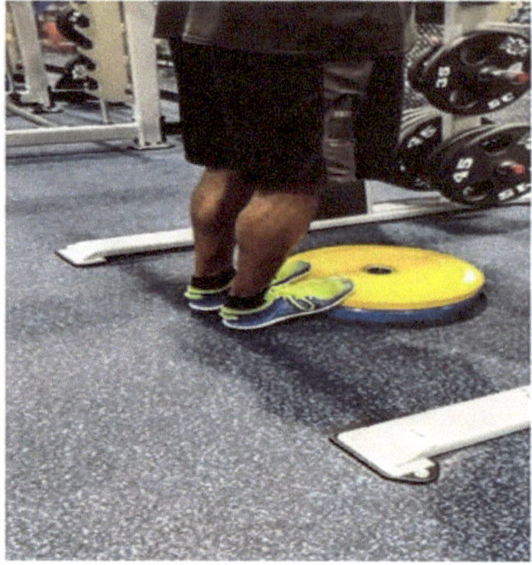

One of my go to's for calf development is the Smith Machine Calf Raise. Notice the picture on the left where he has a full extension at the top of the move and a deep stretch at the bottom of the movement. Many ways to do this move to up the difficulty level, like one foot at a time, heavier weights, pausing at the top or everyone's favorite, just repping it out. Calves is another one of those muscles that's troublesome to grow, but with a lot of reps, frequency, and attention to detail, you can get it done. Spend a lot of time squeezing the blood through your muscles at the top of the movement, typically holding for 3 secs before lowering back down to a full stretch.

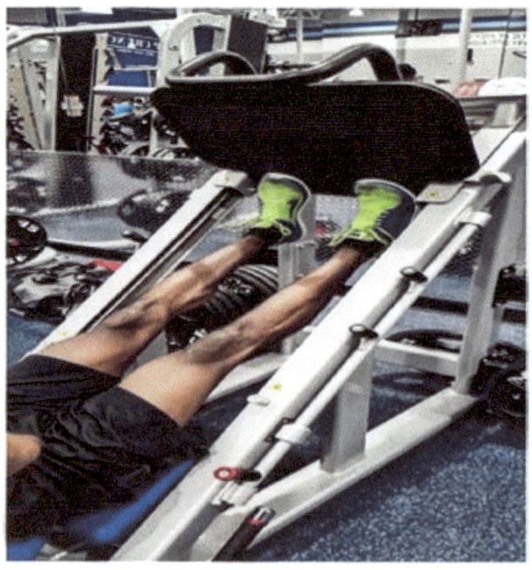 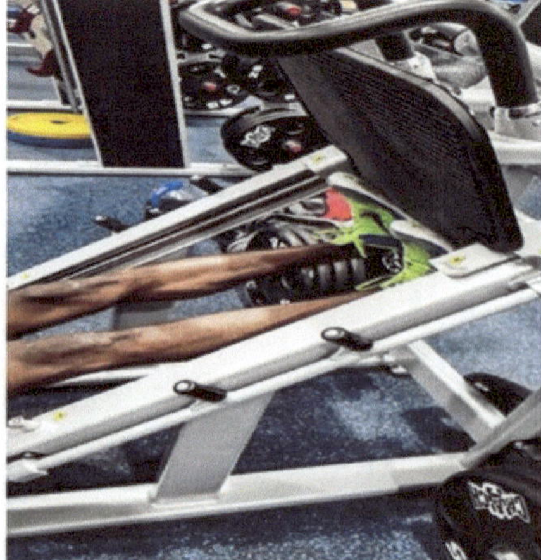

Using the leg press for calves is my go-to for just trying to get as many reps in as I can by doing triple drop sets per set. Typically going from heavy for 8-12 reps to light for 12-15reps for 2 sets. Again focusing on full range of motion. To really step up the intensity, do raise calf raises in between dropping the weight without stopping for a guaanteed burn.

Calf raises <u>are done</u>, one leg at a time. Go up as high as you possibly can, squeezing hard on the calf muscle for each rep. After that, go to a full-down position to full stretch the muscle. Once you do the last rep of your legs, use both feet using the same weight to finish another five to 10 reps for the movement. Hold this for three seconds, ensuring that the calves have <u>been squeezed</u>.

Other Movements You Can Do:

- Donkey Calf Raise

- Leg Press

- Seated Leg Curls

MOVEMENTS FOR SHOULDERS

Shoulders use to be a weak point for me which caused me to get creative with my shoulder workouts. These movements have been a staple in my shoulder program for years, and I know that if applied right, you can see some major growth as I have.

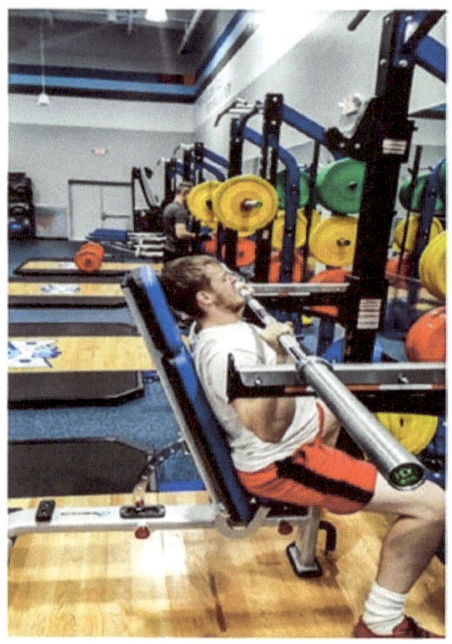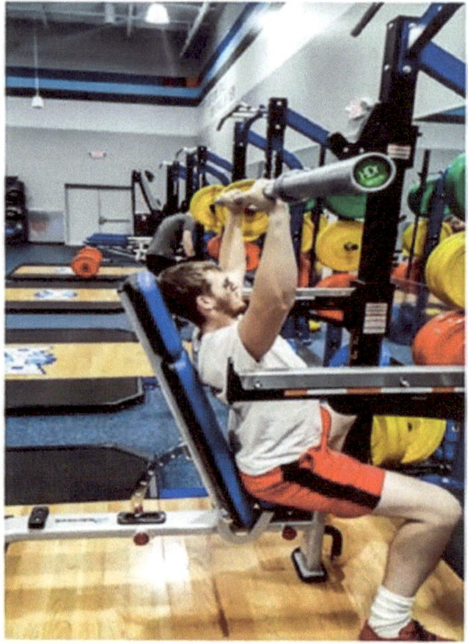

SHOULDER SECRETS #1: This variation of the sitting shoulder press focuses on training for strength. As you can see, the starting point is at 90 degrees. The goal is not to rep it out as you would in a regular bodybuilding scheme, but to explode to top position, pause for 3 seconds (one one thousand..two one thousand, etc) then lower in a slowly controlled manor. Pausing at the bottom of the movement for again 3 seconds before exploding to the top again.

Sample workout: 3-5 reps moderate heavy weight for 3-5 sets

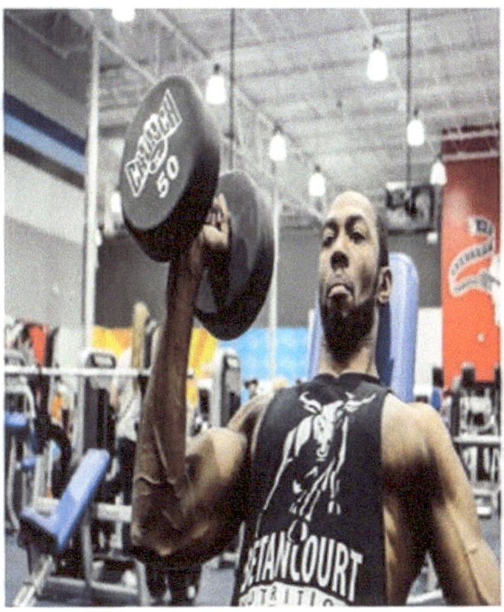 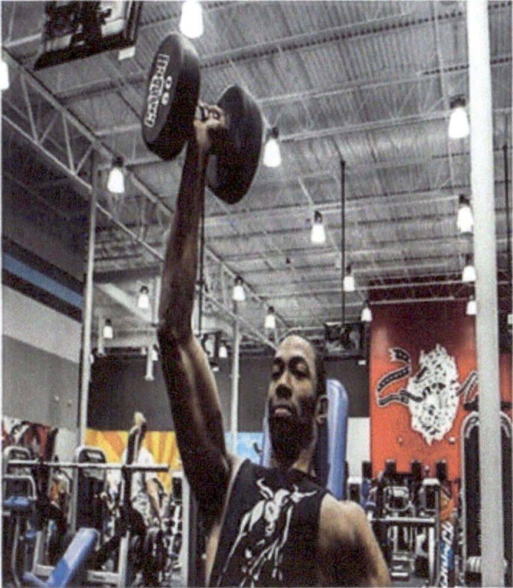

<u>SHOULDER SECRET #2:</u> Another variation of the shoulder press is the seated unilateral shoulder press, focusing on one side at a time to make sure that both sides get an equal amount of work.

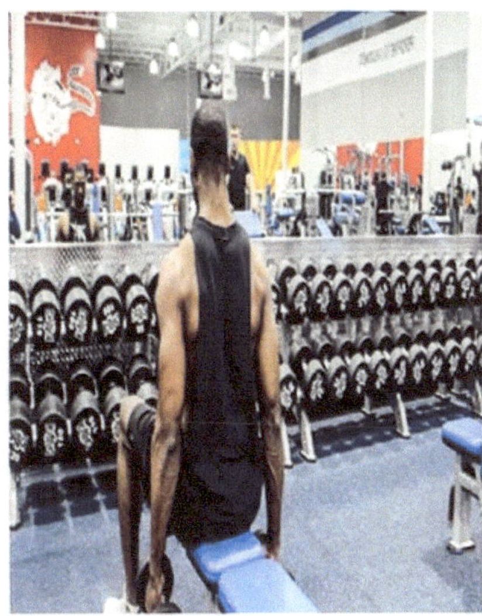 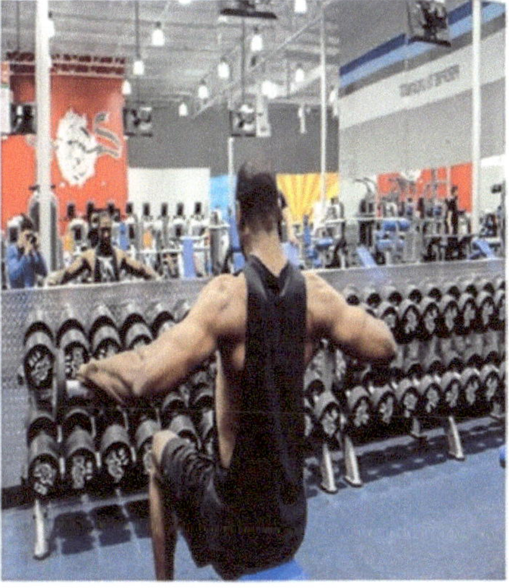

<u>SHOULDER SECRETS #3:</u> With the lateral side raise, a lot of people do this move with almost straight arms and look like they are trying to flap away. The secret is to lead with the elbows and contract the shoulder blades. By doing this, you hit your traps as a byproduct of doing this, killing two birds with one stone.

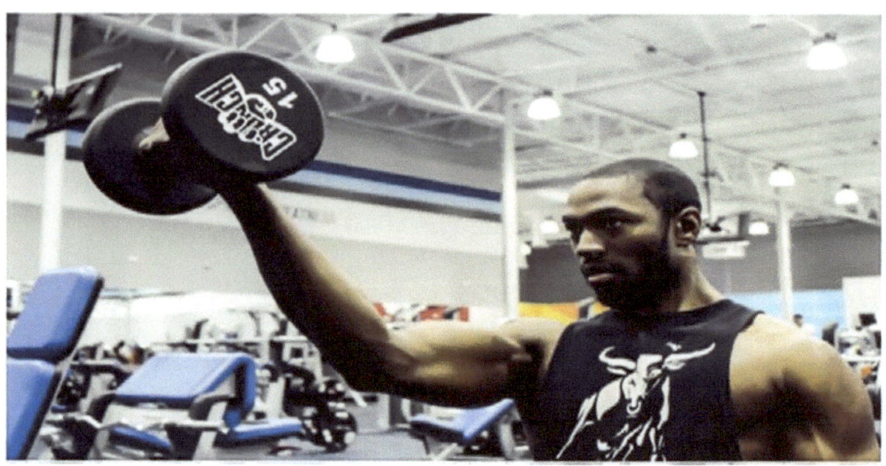

<u>SHOULDER SECRET #4:</u> Notice how both of these movements is sitting down. The goal is to build strength in both shoulders equally. The secret to this move is as you come up, cross the center line of your body to hit the front delt and the small piece of muscle between the chest and shoulder in one smooth motion.

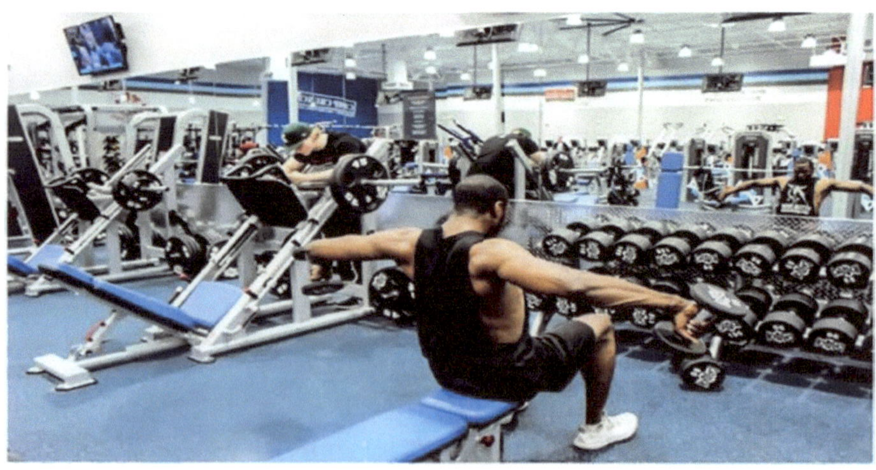

When it comes to the standing shoulder press, you've got two ways in which you can complete the exercise. Run the rack or pick five different sized weights and hit all of them five times until you reach the heaviest dumbbell weight. Now, you can quit upon reaching the heaviest weight or go back down the rack, three times.

With the other back exercises, you do them until you complete the last rep in the standing upright rows... no resting allowed!

Other Movements You Can Do:

- Front Raises with Easy Curl Bar (bring your elbows together

- Standing Shoulder Press

- Seated Shoulder Press

So now that you're armed with the knowledge to complete these moves efficiently let's get to the fun part, the WORKOUT PLAN! I set up the training split as one muscle a day, 5 days on 2 days off to focus on each muscle individually. But you can set up your training split to what works best for you inter-changing the movements from week to week. All of the workouts focus around the 3 main lifts, Bench Press, Deadlift, and Squat, and if I might add, Shoulder Press. Everything after these lifts is all supplement movements to shape the muscles to our desires. The Ab workout will be done before your main workout 3 days a week every other day. Calves are done on the other days.

Monday-Legs

Warm-up*- Static Stretching 2-4 mins*

Slow body weight squats 20 reps

Hanging Leg Raise *(front)Superset with* ***Hanging Leg Raise*** *(side) 10-20 reps per side 3 rounds*

Squat*-(heavyweight) 5x5 superset with single leg press (moderate weight) for 8-12 reps*

Rest 90 secs.

Leg Extensions*- Pyramid style going from light (10 reps each) to heavy (5 reps each) for 1 set then going in the reverse order for the 2nd set.*

Rest 90 secs.

Lying Leg Curls/Seated Leg Curls*- 8-12 reps (moderate weight) superset with stiff leg dead lifts 8-12 reps (moderate weight) 3 sets*

Rest 90 secs.

Smith Machine Calf Raise/Leg Press Calf Extensions*- 15-20 reps (moderate-heavy weight) 3-4 sets*

Rest 90 secs.

Tuesday-Back

Smith Machine Calf Raise*-15-20 reps (moderate weight) 4 sets*

Warm-up*- Pull-ups- 5-10 reps 2 sets*

Deadlift*- Deadlift/Rack pulls 3-4 sets of 8-12 reps superset with Single Arm Dumbbell Row 8-12 reps*

Pull-Ups*- 3 sets 5-10 reps*

Lat Pull-Down*- 3 Rounds of two drop sets (1st set 8 reps, 2nd set 10-12 reps, and 3rd set 12 to 15 reps... resting period for 90 seconds)*

Pull-Ups*- 3 sets 5-10 reps*

Less than 2 minute resting period

Wednesday-Chest

Hanging Leg Raise (front)*Superset with* *Hanging Leg Raise* *(side) 10-20 reps per side 3 rounds*

Warm-Up-Push-Ups – three sets for eight to 10 reps

Incline Bench Press – three to four sets, eight to 12 reps (moderate-heavy weight)

Superset with Decline machine press – three to four sets (light-moderate weight)

Cable Crossovers – three to four sets, five to 10 reps (light weight with a focus on squeezing at the top of the movement)

No more than two minutes rest

Thursday-Shoulders

Leg Press Calf Extensions- *15-20 reps (moderate-heavy weight) 3-4 sets*

Warm-Up- *Shoulder press 15-20 reps 2 sets (lightweight)*

Standing Dumbbell Shoulder Press *- run the rack three to four rounds)*

Seated Lateral Side Raises *- three to four sets, eight to 12 reps*

Seated Lateral Front Raise *– three to four sets, eight to 12 reps*

Superset with Standing Upright Rows – three to four sets, five to eight reps

Rest for no more than two minutes

Friday-Arms

Hanging Leg Raise (front)Superset with *Hanging Leg Raise* (side) 10-20 reps per side 3 rounds

Warm-ups- Curls two sets of 15 to 20 reps (light weight)

Standing Alternating Dumbbell Curls- (three to four rounds) - Biceps

Incline Dumbbell Curls- (three to four sets of drops sets) 8 to 15 reps (moderate weight)

Cable Kickbacks- three sets of 8 to 10 reps (moderate weight)

Straight Bar Pull Down- running stack for two to three rounds – Triceps

Rest – 1 to 2 minutes